# GASTROPARESIS

# cookbook for

## *Beginners*

*Over 100 Delicious Recipes for Digestive Wellbeing to Managing, healing and treating Gastroparesis| 30 day meal plan for managing nausea, quick pain relief and acid reflux*

## Dr. Benjamin Thompson

# Copyright © [2024] by [Dr. Benjamin Thompson]



This book is designed to provide information about **Gastroparesis cookbook for beginners**. The content is intended for educational purposes and is not a substitute for professional medical advice, diagnosis, or treatment. Always seek the advice of your physician or qualified health provider regarding any medical condition or before starting any fitness program.

The author and publisher of this book have made reasonable efforts to ensure the accuracy of the information provided. However, they disclaim responsibility for any liability, loss, or risk, personal or otherwise, which is incurred as a consequence, directly or indirectly, of the use and application of any of the contents of this book.

Any reference to specific exercises, techniques, or nutritional advice is intended for informational purposes only and may not be suitable for every individual. Readers are encouraged to consult with qualified fitness professionals or healthcare providers before initiating any exercise program or dietary changes.

While every effort has been made to provide current and up-to-date information, the author and publisher do not guarantee the accuracy, completeness, or timeliness of the content presented in this book

# TABLE OF CONTENT

## 2.4 Gastroparesis-Friendly Snack and Dessert Recipes ------- 125

# 30 DAYS GASTROPARESIS MEAL PLAN

**W**elcome to your personalized 30-day journey toward managing gastroparesis through gentle and nourishing meals. This meal plan has been carefully crafted to provide you with a variety of stomach-friendly breakfasts, lunches, and dinners. Each day, you'll experience a blend of flavors and textures that are not just kind to your stomach but also packed with essential nutrients.

Throughout this meal plan, you'll find a range of recipes designed to be gentle on your digestion while ensuring a balanced and satisfying diet. From soft and comforting breakfast porridges to flavorful stir-fries and casseroles, every meal has been thoughtfully curated to provide you with both nourishment and ease.

Further into this cookbook, each meal will be further elaborated upon, guiding you through the detailed ingredients, cooking procedures, and nutritional information. Dive into a world of delicious, gastroparesis-friendly recipes designed to make your journey to healthier eating both manageable and enjoyable.

Enjoy your the comprehensive cookbook, where each meal will be meticulously explained, helping you navigate your culinary journey toward managing gastroparesis with ease and flavor.

## Day 1:

- **Breakfast:** Soft Berry Oatmeal
- **Lunch:** Soft Turkey Wrap
- **Dinner:** Soft Chicken and Vegetable Stir-Fry

## Day 2:

- **Breakfast:** Soft Banana Pancakes
- **Lunch:** Soft Tuna Salad
- **Dinner:** Soft Eggplant and Tomato Bake

## Day 3:

- **Breakfast:** Soft Scrambled Eggs with Spinach
- **Lunch:** Soft Lentil Soup
- **Dinner:** Soft Chicken and Broccoli Casserole

## Day 4:

- **Breakfast:** Soft Apple Cinnamon Porridge
- **Lunch:** Soft Turkey and Brown Rice Pilaf
- **Dinner:** Soft Beef and Mushroom Stroganoff

## Day 5:

- **Breakfast:** Soft Yogurt Parfait
- **Lunch:** Soft Chicken Salad
- **Dinner:** Soft Egg Drop Stir-Fry

## Day 6:

- **Breakfast:** Soft Quinoa Breakfast Bowl
- **Lunch:** Soft Turkey and Sweet Potato Mash
- **Dinner:** Soft Chicken and Cauliflower Rice

## Day 7:

- **Breakfast:** Soft Pumpkin Spice Smoothie
- **Lunch:** Soft Chicken and Rice Soup
- **Dinner:** Soft Beef and Quinoa Stuffed Peppers

## Day 8:

- **Breakfast:** Soft Blueberry Chia Pudding
- **Lunch:** Soft Chicken Caesar Salad
- **Dinner:** Soft Chicken and Spinach Pasta

## Day 9:

- **Breakfast:** Soft Mango Smoothie Bowl
- **Lunch:** Soft Turkey and Vegetable Stir-Fry
- **Dinner:** Soft Turkey and Rice Casserole

## Day 10:

- **Breakfast:** Soft Apple Almond Butter Toast
- **Lunch:** Soft Lentil and Vegetable Curry
- **Dinner:** Soft Chicken and Zucchini Bake

## Day 11:

- **Breakfast:** Soft Avocado Toast
- **Lunch:** Soft Beef and Potato Soup
- **Dinner:** Soft Turkey and Mushroom Skewers

## Day 12:

- **Breakfast:** Soft Strawberry Banana Yogurt Bowl
- **Lunch:** Soft Chicken and Quinoa Salad
- **Dinner:** Soft Chicken and Rice Pilaf

**Day 13:**

- **Breakfast:** Soft Pear and Cinnamon Oatmeal
- **Lunch:** Soft Tuna and Brown Rice Salad
- **Dinner:** Soft Beef and Bell Pepper Stir-Fry

**Day 14:**

- **Breakfast:** Soft Greek Yogurt Parfait
- **Lunch:** Soft Chicken and Rice Soup
- **Dinner:** Soft Beef and Eggplant Bake

**Day 15:**

- **Breakfast:** Soft Banana Oat Cookies
- **Lunch:** Soft Lentil Soup
- **Dinner:** Soft Chicken and Broccoli Casserole

**Day 16:**

- **Breakfast:** Soft Berry Smoothie Bowl
- **Lunch:** Soft Turkey Wrap
- **Dinner:** Soft Eggplant and Tomato Bake

**Day 17:**

- **Breakfast:** Soft Baked Apples
- **Lunch:** Soft Chicken Salad
- **Dinner:** Soft Beef and Mushroom Stroganoff

**Day 18:**

- **Breakfast:** Soft Yogurt Parfait
- **Lunch:** Soft Tuna Salad
- **Dinner:** Soft Chicken and Cauliflower Rice

## Day 19:

- **Breakfast:** Soft Pumpkin Pudding
- **Lunch:** Soft Chicken Caesar Salad
- **Dinner:** Soft Egg Drop Stir-Fry

## Day 20:

- **Breakfast:** Soft Chia Seed Pudding
- **Lunch:** Soft Turkey and Sweet Potato Mash
- **Dinner:** Soft Chicken and Zucchini Bake

## Day 21:

- **Breakfast:** Soft Baked Pear with Cinnamon
- **Lunch:** Soft Turkey and Brown Rice Pilaf
- **Dinner:** Soft Turkey and Rice Casserole

## Day 22:

- **Breakfast:** Soft Blueberry Chia Jam on Toast
- **Lunch:** Soft Chicken and Quinoa Salad
- **Dinner:** Soft Beef and Bell Pepper Stir-Fry

## Day 23:

- **Breakfast:** Soft Chocolate Chia Pudding
- **Lunch:** Soft Turkey and Vegetable Stir-Fry
- **Dinner:** Soft Chicken and Spinach Pasta

## Day 24:

- **Breakfast:** Soft Rice Cake with Cottage Cheese and Berries
- **Lunch:** Soft Lentil and Vegetable Curry
- **Dinner:** Soft Chicken and Rice Pilaf

## Day 25:

- **Breakfast:** Soft Mango Yogurt Popsicles
- **Lunch:** Soft Turkey Wrap
- **Dinner:** Soft Beef and Quinoa Stuffed Peppers

## Day 26:

- **Breakfast:** Soft Avocado Chocolate Mousse
- **Lunch:** Soft Tuna and Brown Rice Salad
- **Dinner:** Soft Chicken and Rice Soup

## Day 27:

- **Breakfast:** Soft Banana Pancakes
- **Lunch:** Soft Chicken Salad
- **Dinner:** Soft Eggplant and Tomato Bake

## Day 28:

- **Breakfast:** Soft Peanut Butter and Jelly Sandwiches
- **Lunch:** Soft Beef and Potato Soup
- **Dinner:** Soft Turkey and Mushroom Skewers

## Day 29:

- **Breakfast:** Soft Apple Cinnamon Porridge
- **Lunch:** Soft Lentil Soup
- **Dinner:** Soft Chicken and Broccoli Casserole

## Day 30:

- **Breakfast:** Soft Berry Smoothie Bowl
- **Lunch:** Soft Turkey Wrap
- **Dinner:** Soft Eggplant and Tomato Bake

# ABOUT THE AUTHOR

**D**r. Benjamin Thompson *stands at the forefront of healthcare innovation, with a career spanning decades dedicated to healing, research, and redefining the boundaries of holistic wellness. A trailblazer in oncology and disease management, Dr. Thompson's profound expertise and unwavering dedication have transformed countless lives.*

Dr. Thompson embarked on his journey as a beacon of hope in the realm of healthcare, earning his medical degree with honors from a prestigious institution. His insatiable curiosity and commitment to patient-centric care led him into the intricate world of oncology and disease management.

**Pioneering Breakthroughs:**

Throughout his illustrious career, Dr. Thompson spearheaded groundbreaking research initiatives, pioneering advancements in cancer treatment modalities and disease management strategies. His relentless pursuit of excellence and innovation resulted in several patented methodologies and groundbreaking protocols for disease intervention.

Renowned for his expertise in navigating the complexities of cancer and chronic diseases, Dr. Thompson's contributions to the medical field have earned him widespread recognition and accolades. His comprehensive approach to patient care encompasses cutting-edge treatments, compassionate support, and a profound understanding of the holistic aspects of healing.

## Transition to Culinary Solutions:

Driven by a vision to expand healing beyond traditional medical boundaries, Dr. Thompson embarked on a transformative journey. Leveraging his extensive knowledge of health and nutrition, he transitioned into crafting innovative cookbooks aimed at addressing life's health challenges through culinary solutions.

## Cookbooks as Healing Tools:

Dr. Thompson's culinary masterpieces transcend the realm of conventional cookbooks. Each meticulously crafted recipe is a testament to his deep-rooted belief in the healing potential of food. His cookbooks seamlessly integrate medical expertise with culinary artistry, offering not just meals but transformative solutions to alleviate health struggles.

## Empowering Health through Food:

With an unwavering commitment to empowering individuals in their health journeys, Dr. Thompson's cookbooks serve as invaluable guides. They encapsulate not only delectable recipes but also evidence-based strategies to manage health conditions, elevate well-being, and embrace a nourishing lifestyle.

## Personal Journey and Vision:

Dr. Benjamin Thompson's professional accomplishments are not just a testament to his expertise but a reflection of a life dedicated to enhancing the human experience. His relentless pursuit of innovative solutions and compassionate care continues to inspire hope and redefine the paradigm of health and healing.

Dr. Thompson's life's work exemplifies a harmonious blend of medical expertise, culinary mastery, and an unwavering commitment to enhancing lives. His cookbooks stand as a testament to his vision: transforming meals into pathways for healing and embracing a life of vitality and wellness.

# INTRODUCTION

I n the quiet hum of a bustling kitchen, where aromas dance and pots simmer, there exists a world where food transcends mere sustenance. It's a world where every meal is an act of resilience, a celebration of adaptation, and a testament to the unwavering spirit of those touched by gastroparesis.

Imagine sitting down to a meal, your anticipation tinged with uncertainty, your hunger mingled with caution. This is the reality for countless individuals navigating the labyrinth of gastroparesis, a condition that disrupts the rhythm of digestion and redefines the relationship with food.

Within these pages lies more than just a collection of recipes; it's a narrative woven with empathy, resilience, and the collective experiences of a community united by a shared journey. Let me introduce you to Mia.

Mia's journey began with a diagnosis that altered the very fabric of her daily life. Faced with the challenges of gastroparesis, she embarked on a quest to redefine her culinary world. What initially felt like a maze of limitations soon transformed into an adventure of creativity and nourishment. Through trial and error, tears and triumphs, Mia discovered the art of crafting meals that nurtured both body and soul.

Her kitchen became a sanctuary, a canvas where she painted with flavors, textures, and care. Each recipe was a testament to her resilience, a melody composed amidst the symphony of gastric delays. But Mia's story is not hers alone; it's a reflection of countless individuals maneuvering through the nuances of gastroparesis.

As you embark on this culinary expedition, know that each recipe, each tip, and each insight shared here is imbued with empathy and understanding. It's a guidebook crafted not just with expertise but with a heartfelt desire to empower and uplift.

So, whether you're a newcomer to the realm of gastroparesis or a seasoned traveler along this path, may this cookbook be your trusted companion. May it transform your kitchen into a realm of possibilities, where nourishment transcends challenges and each bite is savored with gratitude.

Welcome to a world where food isn't just sustenance; it's a celebration of resilience. Welcome to "Savoring Every Bite: Nourishing Your Journey Through Gastroparesis."

# *how common is gastroparesis*

Gastroparesis, though not as widely recognized as some other gastrointestinal conditions, is more common than many might think. Understanding its prevalence helps shed light on its impact and the number of individuals affected by this condition.

## How Common is Gastroparesis?

Gastroparesis, while not considered rare, is not always easily diagnosed or reported. The prevalence of gastroparesis in the general population is estimated to be approximately 0.2% to 2% worldwide. However, these figures might be underestimates due to several factors:

## 1. Underdiagnosis and Misdiagnosis:

- **Symptom Variability:** Symptoms of gastroparesis can vary widely and overlap with other digestive disorders, leading to misdiagnosis or delayed diagnosis.

- **Diagnostic Challenges:** Diagnostic tests for gastroparesis are not always performed unless symptoms are severe or persistent, contributing to underdiagnosis.

## 2. Underreporting and Lack of Awareness:

- **Misunderstanding of Symptoms:** Mild symptoms might be attributed to other issues or might be overlooked, leading to underreporting.

- **Lack of Awareness:** Many people might not recognize the symptoms of gastroparesis or might not seek medical attention for mild symptoms, contributing to underreporting in statistics.

## 3. Associated Conditions and Risk Factors:

- **Diabetes:** Gastroparesis is more commonly reported among individuals with diabetes. Roughly 30% to 40% of people with Type 1 or Type 2 diabetes may experience gastroparesis symptoms.

- **Other Health Conditions:** Conditions such as autoimmune disorders, neurological diseases, and post-surgical complications can increase the risk of gastroparesis.

## 4. Impact on Quality of Life:

- **Varied Severity:** Symptoms of gastroparesis can range from mild inconvenience to severe disruption of daily life. Many individuals might cope with mild symptoms without seeking medical attention.

## 5. Demographic Factors:

- **Gender and Age:** Some studies suggest gastroparesis might be more common in women than in men. It can affect individuals of any age but is more frequently diagnosed in adults.

While statistics might not fully capture the prevalence of gastroparesis due to underdiagnosis, underreporting, and the complexity of its symptoms, it's evident that this condition affects a significant number of individuals globally. Improved awareness among healthcare providers, increased recognition of symptoms, and better diagnostic tools can contribute to a more accurate understanding of the true prevalence of gastroparesis.

Enhancing understanding, early diagnosis, and targeted management strategies are crucial in providing better support and improving the quality of life for those living with gastroparesis.

# Chapter 1: Understanding Gastroparesis

## 1.1 Introduction to Gastroparesis

### Overview of Gastroparesis: Causes, symptoms, and diagnosis

**Causes of Gastroparesis:**

Gastroparesis is primarily a disorder of the digestive system, characterized by delayed emptying of the stomach. While the exact cause isn't always clear, several factors can contribute:

- **Nerve Damage:** A prevalent cause is damage to the vagus nerve, responsible for controlling the muscles of the stomach. This damage can result from surgery, injury, or conditions like diabetes.

- **Viral Infections:** Certain infections, particularly viral ones, can affect the nerves controlling stomach muscles, leading to gastroparesis.

- **Medications:** Some medications, such as certain antidepressants and high blood pressure drugs, may contribute to delayed gastric emptying.

- **Smooth Muscle Disorders:** Conditions affecting the smooth muscles of the stomach can impede normal contractions needed for digestion.

- **Other Health Conditions:** Diseases like Parkinson's, multiple sclerosis, and autoimmune disorders may indirectly lead to gastroparesis.

**Symptoms of Gastroparesis:**

Recognizing the symptoms of gastroparesis is crucial for early intervention and management:

- **Nausea and Vomiting:** Persistent feelings of nausea and vomiting, especially after eating, are common symptoms.

- **Feeling Full Quickly:** Individuals with gastroparesis often feel full even after consuming small amounts of food.

- **Abdominal Pain:** Discomfort or pain in the abdominal region may accompany delayed stomach emptying.

- **Bloating:** Excessive gas and bloating are frequent symptoms, contributing to abdominal discomfort.

- **Changes in Blood Sugar Levels:** For individuals with diabetes, managing blood sugar levels can become challenging due to unpredictable digestion.

- **Unexplained Weight Loss:** In severe cases, gastroparesis can lead to unintended weight loss.

## Diagnosis of Gastroparesis:

Diagnosing gastroparesis involves a combination of clinical evaluation, medical history assessment, and diagnostic tests:

- **Medical History and Physical Examination:** Healthcare professionals will inquire about symptoms, medical history, and conduct a physical examination to assess abdominal tenderness and bloating.

- **Blood Tests:** Blood tests can help identify underlying conditions, including diabetes or infections, which may contribute to gastroparesis.

- **Imaging Studies:** Tests like upper gastrointestinal (GI) series or abdominal ultrasound may be conducted to visualize the stomach and rule out other issues.

- **Gastric Emptying Study:** This is a key diagnostic test where the patient consumes a meal containing a small amount of radioactive material. Imaging scans then track the movement of the material through the digestive tract, highlighting any delays.

- **Electrogastrography (EGG):** This test measures the electrical activity of the stomach muscles and can help identify abnormalities in contractions.

- **Endoscopy:** In some cases, an endoscopy may be performed to examine the stomach lining and rule out other digestive disorders.

## Impact on digestion and daily life

**Disrupted Digestive Process:**

Gastroparesis significantly disrupts the normal digestive process, impacting the breakdown and movement of food through the gastrointestinal tract:

- **Delayed Stomach Emptying:** One of the hallmark features of gastroparesis is the slowed movement of food from the stomach into the small intestine. This delay can result in prolonged feelings of fullness and discomfort after eating.

- **Impaired Nutrient Absorption:** Slower digestion can affect the body's ability to absorb nutrients, leading to deficiencies in essential vitamins and minerals, despite consuming a balanced diet.

## 2. Dietary Challenges and Nutritional Impact:

Managing a proper diet becomes a crucial aspect of coping with gastroparesis:

- **Limited Food Choices:** Individuals with gastroparesis often need to modify their diet, opting for easily digestible, low-fiber foods to reduce the risk of complications such as blockages or discomfort.

- **Balancing Nutritional Needs:** Meeting daily nutritional requirements can become challenging due to dietary restrictions. Patients may struggle to obtain sufficient calories and essential nutrients, leading to potential weight loss or malnutrition.

## 3. Impact on Eating Patterns:

Gastroparesis can significantly alter an individual's eating habits and meal schedules:

- **Frequent Small Meals:** Eating smaller, more frequent meals can help manage symptoms by reducing the volume of food in the stomach at any given time, aiding digestion.

- **Meal Planning Challenges:** Planning meals becomes more complex as individuals need to balance nutritional needs with foods that are easier to digest, often requiring careful preparation and consideration.

## 4. Effects on Daily Activities and Quality of Life:

Gastroparesis can have broader implications on a person's daily life beyond eating habits:

- **Social and Emotional Impact:** Coping with a chronic digestive disorder can lead to emotional distress, impacting social interactions, mental health, and overall well-being.

- **Fatigue and Energy Levels:** Digestive issues and nutritional deficiencies can contribute to fatigue and reduced energy levels, affecting productivity and daily activities.

- **Work and Productivity:** Managing symptoms, dietary needs, and potential fatigue can affect work performance and productivity, necessitating adjustments and accommodations.

## 5. Medical Management and Lifestyle Adjustments:

Effective management of gastroparesis requires a combination of medical interventions and lifestyle adjustments:

- **Medications:** Some patients may benefit from medications that help stimulate stomach contractions or manage symptoms like nausea and vomiting.

- **Dietary Modifications:** Working closely with a dietitian to develop personalized meal plans can aid in symptom management and ensure adequate nutrition.

- **Lifestyle Changes:** Adopting stress management techniques, engaging in gentle exercises, and prioritizing self-care can contribute to symptom alleviation and better overall health.

## 6. Healthcare and Support Networks:

Access to healthcare professionals and support networks is crucial for individuals managing gastroparesis:

- **Medical Monitoring:** Regular check-ups, monitoring of symptoms, and adjustments in treatment plans are essential for effective disease management.

- **Support Groups:** Engaging with support groups or connecting with others facing similar challenges can provide emotional support, share coping strategies, and offer valuable insights into managing gastroparesis.

# *1.2 Managing Gastroparesis*

## Dietary guidelines for gastroparesis

Gastroparesis presents unique challenges in the realm of diet and nutrition, necessitating a thoughtful and tailored approach to food choices. Understanding the impact of various foods on digestion and adopting strategies to alleviate symptoms are pivotal in managing this condition and enhancing overall well-being.

### 1. Understanding Gastroparesis and its Impact on Diet:

Gastroparesis, characterized by delayed gastric emptying, affects the normal movement of food through the digestive tract. This condition necessitates dietary modifications to ease digestive discomfort and ensure optimal nutrient intake.

### 1.1 Gastroparesis Symptoms and Their Relation to Food Choices:

- **Nausea and Vomiting:** Certain foods might exacerbate these symptoms, while others may help alleviate discomfort.

- **Feeling Full Quickly:** Smaller, more frequent meals with easily digestible foods can prevent excessive fullness.

- **Abdominal Pain and Bloating:** Food choices can impact the severity of these symptoms. Selecting low-fiber, easily digestible options is beneficial.

### 2. Key Principles of a Gastroparesis-Friendly Diet:

### 2.1 Low-Fiber Choices:

Fiber can be challenging to digest and might worsen symptoms. Opt for low-fiber alternatives:

- **Vegetables:** Cooked or canned vegetables without skin or seeds (carrots, green beans).

- **Fruits:** Ripe, peeled fruits (bananas, melons) or canned fruits in their juices.

- **Grains:** Refined grains like white bread, pasta, and rice instead of whole grains.

## 2.2 Lean Protein Sources:

Protein is essential for healing and maintaining muscle mass. Select lean options that are easier to digest:

- **Poultry:** Skinless chicken or turkey.
- **Fish:** Low-fat fish varieties such as cod or haddock.
- **Tofu and Eggs:** Easily digestible protein alternatives.

## 2.3 Low-Fat and Low-Residue Choices:

Fatty and high-residue foods can exacerbate symptoms. Choose low-fat alternatives and avoid high-residue foods:

- **Dairy:** Opt for low-fat or fat-free dairy products.
- **Avoid Fried Foods:** Minimize intake of fried or greasy foods.

## 2.4 Soft and Moist Foods:

Texture plays a crucial role in ease of digestion. Focus on foods that are soft and moist:

- **Soups and Stews:** Well-cooked and pureed soups with easily digestible ingredients.
- **Mashed Potatoes or Sweet Potatoes:** Easily digestible starches.

## 3. Dietary Strategies for Symptom Management:

### 3.1 Portion Control and Meal Frequency:

- **Small, Frequent Meals:** Consuming smaller portions throughout the day can aid digestion.
- **Avoid Large Meals:** Large meals can overwhelm the stomach, leading to discomfort.

### 3.2 Fluid Intake and Timing:

- **Hydration Between Meals:** Sip fluids slowly between meals to avoid feeling overly full.

- **Avoid Drinking During Meals:** Consuming liquids during meals can increase stomach volume.

## 3.3 Meal Timing and Posture:

- **Ideal Meal Times:** Eating when symptoms are milder, such as in the morning or when feeling better.

- **Upright Position:** Sit upright while eating to aid digestion and minimize discomfort.

## 4. Cooking Techniques and Food Preparation:

### 4.1 Blending and Pureeing:

- **Texture Modification:** Blending or pureeing foods can aid digestion, especially for severe cases.

- **Smooth Textures:** Pureed soups, smoothies, and blended meals can be easier to digest.

### 4.2 Selective Food Preparation:

- **Remove Tough Parts:** Peel fruits and vegetables, remove seeds, and trim tough portions.

- **Cook Thoroughly:** Well-cooked and tender foods are easier to digest.

## 5. Customizing Diet Plans and Seeking Professional Guidance:

### 5.1 Consultation with a Dietitian:

- **Individualized Plans:** Registered dietitians can create personalized meal plans to suit individual needs.

- **Monitoring and Adjustments:** Regular consultations help adapt diets as symptoms change.

### 5.2 Keeping a Food Diary:

- **Identifying Triggers:** Maintain a diary to track symptoms and identify specific foods that worsen or alleviate discomfort.

## 6. Meal Ideas and Sample Menus for Gastroparesis:

### 6.1 Sample Breakfast Options:

- **Banana-Oatmeal Smoothie:** Blend ripe banana, cooked oats, and low-fat yogurt.
- **Scrambled Eggs:** Softly cooked scrambled eggs with well-cooked vegetables.

### 6.2 Lunch and Dinner Suggestions:

- **Chicken and Rice Soup:** Pureed soup with shredded chicken and well-cooked rice.
- **Tofu Stir-fry:** Soft tofu with lightly cooked vegetables in a light sauce.

### 6.3 Snack and Dessert Ideas:

- **Applesauce:** Homemade or store-bought unsweetened applesauce.
- **Greek Yogurt:** Low-fat, plain Greek yogurt with blended fruit.

## 7. Factors to Consider and Cautionary Notes:

### 7.1 Individual Variations:

- **Trial and Error:** Foods that work for one person might not suit another. Experiment to find what works best.

### 7.2 Medication and Dietary Interactions:

- **Consult Healthcare Providers:** Discuss dietary changes and potential interactions with medications.

## 8. The Role of Stress and Lifestyle Modifications:

### 8.1 Stress Management:

- **Impact on Symptoms:** Stress can exacerbate symptoms. Engage in stress-reducing activities like meditation or yoga.

### 8.2 Gentle Physical Activity:

- **Promoting Digestion:** Light activities, like walking, can aid digestion and overall well-being.

## 9. Advantages of a Gastroparesis-Friendly Diet:

### 9.1 Enhanced Digestive Comfort:

- **Reduced Symptoms:** Adhering to dietary guidelines can alleviate discomfort associated with gastroparesis.

### 9.2 Improved Quality of Life:

- **Better Nutrition:** Despite restrictions, a well-planned diet can ensure adequate nutrient intake.

## 10. Conclusion: Embracing Dietary Modifications for Gastroparesis Management

Gastroparesis necessitates a nuanced approach to dietary choices, focusing on easily digestible, nutrient-dense options while avoiding triggers that exacerbate symptoms. Customizing meal plans, being mindful of food textures, and consulting healthcare professionals play crucial roles in managing this condition effectively. By embracing dietary modifications and making informed food choices, individuals with gastroparesis can attain greater comfort and improve their quality of life.

## Importance of meal planning and portion control

In the fast-paced rhythm of modern life, the significance of intentional and thoughtful meal planning combined with portion control cannot be overstated. Beyond the realms of weight management, these practices play pivotal roles in fostering overall health, supporting nutritional balance, and contributing to the prevention and management of various health conditions. This comprehensive exploration delves into the multifaceted importance of meal planning and portion control, unraveling their impacts on physical well-being, psychological health, and the broader canvas of sustainable lifestyle choices.

## 1. Nutritional Balance and Wellness:

### 1.1 Strategic Macronutrient Distribution:

- **Energy Requirements:** Meal planning allows for the calculation of daily energy needs, ensuring an appropriate balance of macronutrients—proteins, carbohydrates, and fats.

- **Optimal Functioning:** Proper distribution of macronutrients supports bodily functions, from energy production to immune system activity.

## 1.2 Micronutrient Sufficiency:

- **Vitamins and Minerals:** A well-structured meal plan facilitates the inclusion of a variety of fruits, vegetables, and whole grains, ensuring adequate intake of essential vitamins and minerals.

- **Preventing Deficiencies:** Portion control helps prevent overconsumption, allowing for a diverse and nutrient-rich diet.

## 1.3 Health Conditions and Dietary Requirements:

- **Chronic Conditions:** Individuals with conditions like diabetes or hypertension benefit from meal planning tailored to their specific needs.

- **Balanced Intake:** Portion control becomes crucial in managing conditions where strict control over certain nutrients, such as sodium or carbohydrates, is necessary.

## 2. Weight Management and Body Composition:

## 2.1 Caloric Control:

- **Preventing Overconsumption:** Portion control aids in preventing excessive calorie intake, a cornerstone of weight management.

- **Weight Loss or Maintenance:** Strategic meal planning supports both weight loss and maintenance goals, aligning with individual needs and lifestyle.

## 2.2 Satiety and Hunger Regulation:

- **Balanced Meals:** A well-planned meal, with appropriate portions of protein, fiber, and healthy fats, promotes satiety and regulates hunger cues.

- **Preventing Overeating:** Portion control prevents overindulgence, allowing the body to signal fullness effectively.

## 2.3 Psychological Well-being:

- **Mindful Eating:** Portion control encourages mindful eating, fostering a healthier relationship with food.

- **Reducing Emotional Eating:** Meal planning provides structure, reducing reliance on impulsive or emotional eating.

## 3. Disease Prevention and Management:

### 3.1 Cardiovascular Health:

- **Heart-Friendly Diets:** Meal plans focusing on lean proteins, whole grains, and unsaturated fats contribute to cardiovascular health.

- **Controlling Sodium Intake:** Portion control helps regulate sodium intake, a crucial factor in managing blood pressure.

### 3.2 Type 2 Diabetes:

- **Carbohydrate Management:** Meal planning assists in managing carbohydrate intake, a key consideration for individuals with diabetes.

- **Blood Sugar Control:** Portion control aids in stabilizing blood sugar levels, preventing spikes.

### 3.3 Gastrointestinal Health:

- **Digestive Comfort:** Smaller, well-distributed meals can alleviate symptoms for individuals with conditions like gastroparesis or acid reflux.

- **Balancing Fiber Intake:** Meal planning helps balance fiber intake, promoting digestive health.

## 4. Energy Levels and Performance:

### 4.1 Consistent Energy Supply:

- **Balanced Meals:** Meal planning ensures a consistent supply of energy throughout the day, preventing energy crashes.

- **Enhanced Physical Performance:** Adequate portions of carbohydrates, proteins, and fats support physical activities and overall vitality.

## 4.2 Cognitive Function:

- **Brain-Nourishing Nutrients:** Proper nutrition, achieved through meal planning, supports cognitive function and mental clarity.

- **Blood Sugar Stability:** Portion control aids in stabilizing blood sugar levels, crucial for sustained mental focus.

## 5. Sustainable and Cost-Efficient Eating:

### 5.1 Reducing Food Waste:

- **Planned Ingredients:** Meal planning involves selecting ingredients strategically, reducing the likelihood of excess perishables going unused.

- **Portion Control:** Cooking and consuming appropriate portions minimize leftovers, contributing to sustainability.

### 5.2 Financial Considerations:

- **Efficient Use of Resources:** Meal planning allows for efficient use of groceries, preventing unnecessary expenses.

- **Reducing Impulse Purchases:** Portion control discourages excessive buying, preventing overconsumption and waste.

## 6. Social and Cultural Considerations:

### 6.1 Shared Meals:

- **Inclusive Planning:** Thoughtful meal planning accommodates various dietary preferences and restrictions, fostering inclusivity.

- **Shared Experience:** Controlled portions allow individuals to enjoy communal meals without compromising their health goals.

### 6.2 Celebrations and Occasions:

- **Strategic Indulgence:** Meal planning allows for moderation during special occasions, preventing excessive consumption.

- **Mindful Celebrations:** Portion control encourages individuals to savor special foods in a mindful and balanced manner.

# Chapter 2: Gastroparesis-Friendly Recipes

## 2.1 Breakfast Options

### 1. Banana Oat Pancakes

**Ingredients:**

- 1 ripe banana
- 1/2 cup rolled oats
- 1 egg
- Cinnamon (optional)
- Cooking spray or oil for pan

**Procedure:**

1. Mash the banana in a bowl and mix in oats and egg.
2. Add a pinch of cinnamon if desired.
3. Heat a pan over medium heat and lightly coat with cooking spray or oil.
4. Pour small portions of the batter onto the pan, cooking until bubbles form, then flipping to cook the other side.
5. Serve warm.

**Nutritional Content (per serving):**

- Calories: 200
- Protein: 7g
- Carbohydrates: 30g
- Fat: 6g
- Fiber: 4g

# 2. Scrambled Tofu

## *Ingredients*:

- 1/2 block of firm tofu, crumbled
- 1/4 cup chopped bell peppers
- 1/4 cup chopped spinach
- 1 tablespoon olive oil
- Salt and pepper to taste

## *Procedure*:

1. Heat olive oil in a pan over medium heat.
2. Add tofu, bell peppers, and spinach.
3. Cook until vegetables are tender and tofu is slightly golden.
4. Season with salt and pepper.
5. Serve warm.

## *Nutritional Content (per serving):*

- Calories: 180
- Protein: 14g
- Carbohydrates: 6g
- Fat: 11g
- Fiber: 2g

# 3. Creamy Banana Smoothie Bowl

## *Ingredients:*

- 1 ripe banana
- 1/2 cup Greek yogurt
- 1/4 cup almond milk
- Toppings: sliced banana, chia seeds, shredded coconut (optional)

## *Procedure:*

1. Blend the ripe banana, Greek yogurt, and almond milk until smooth.
2. Pour the mixture into a bowl.
3. Top with sliced banana, chia seeds, and shredded coconut if desired.
4. Serve chilled.

## *Nutritional Content (per serving):*

- Calories: 220
- Protein: 14g
- Carbohydrates: 30g
- Fat: 6g
- Fiber: 5g

## 4. Quinoa Breakfast Bowl

### *Ingredients:*

- 1/2 cup cooked quinoa
- 1/4 cup blueberries
- 1 tablespoon honey
- 1 tablespoon chopped nuts (almonds, walnuts)
- Splash of almond milk (optional)

### *Procedure:*

1. In a bowl, layer cooked quinoa, blueberries, and chopped nuts.
2. Drizzle honey over the top.
3. Add a splash of almond milk if desired.
4. Mix well before eating.

### *Nutritional Content (per serving):*

- Calories: 250
- Protein: 8g
- Carbohydrates: 40g
- Fat: 7g
- Fiber: 6g

## 5. Egg and Spinach Wrap

**Ingredients:**

- 2 eggs
- 1/4 cup chopped spinach
- 1 whole grain tortilla
- Salt and pepper to taste

**Procedure:**

1. Scramble eggs in a pan over medium heat.
2. Add chopped spinach to the eggs and cook until wilted.
3. Season with salt and pepper.
4. Place the egg and spinach mixture in a whole grain tortilla and wrap.
5. Serve warm.

**Nutritional Content (per serving):**

- Calories: 280
- Protein: 15g
- Carbohydrates: 20g
- Fat: 12g
- Fiber: 5g

# 6. Chia Seed Pudding

## *Ingredients:*

- 2 tablespoons chia seeds
- 1/2 cup almond milk
- 1/4 teaspoon vanilla extract
- Fresh berries for topping

## *Procedure:*

1. Mix chia seeds, almond milk, and vanilla extract in a bowl.
2. Stir well and let it sit for 10 minutes, stirring occasionally.
3. Refrigerate overnight or until the mixture thickens to a pudding-like consistency.
4. Top with fresh berries before serving.

## *Nutritional Content (per serving):*

- Calories: 150
- Protein: 5g
- Carbohydrates: 15g
- Fat: 8g
- Fiber: 9g

## 7. Cinnamon Apple Porridge

*Ingredients:*

- 1/2 cup cooked oatmeal
- 1/2 apple, diced
- 1/4 teaspoon cinnamon
- 1 teaspoon honey

*Procedure*:

1. Mix cooked oatmeal with diced apple and cinnamon.
2. Warm the mixture in a saucepan until the apple softens.
3. Drizzle honey on top before serving.

*Nutritional Content (per serving):*

- Calories: 210
- Protein: 5g
- Carbohydrates: 40g
- Fat: 3g
- Fiber: 6g

## 8. Soft-Boiled Eggs with Toast Soldiers

*Ingredients:*

- 2 eggs
- 2 slices of white bread, toasted and sliced into strips
- Salt and pepper to taste

*Procedure:*

1. Boil the eggs for 4-5 minutes for a soft-boiled consistency.
2. Serve with toasted bread strips (soldiers) for dipping.
3. Season with salt and pepper to taste.

*Nutritional Content (per serving):*

- Calories: 240
- Protein: 12g
- Carbohydrates: 25g
- Fat: 10g
- Fiber: 2g

# 9. Yogurt Parfait

## *Ingredients:*

- 1/2 cup plain Greek yogurt
- 1/4 cup granola
- 1/4 cup mixed berries
- 1 tablespoon honey (optional)

## *Procedure:*

1. Layer Greek yogurt, granola, and mixed berries in a glass or bowl.
2. Drizzle honey on top if desired.
3. Serve chilled.

## *Nutritional Content (per serving):*

- Calories: 260
- Protein: 15g
- Carbohydrates: 35g
- Fat: 7g
- Fiber: 5g

# 10. Peanut Butter Banana Toast

## *Ingredients:*

- 1 slice whole grain bread, toasted
- 1 tablespoon peanut butter
- 1/2 banana, sliced

## *Procedure*:

1. Spread peanut butter on the toasted bread.
2. Arrange banana slices on top.
3. Enjoy as an open-faced sandwich.

## *Nutritional Content (per serving):*

- Calories: 280
- Protein: 8g
- Carbohydrates: 30g
- Fat: 15g
- Fiber: 5g

# 11. Rice Pudding with Cinnamon

## *Ingredients:*

- 1/2 cup cooked white rice
- 1/2 cup almond milk
- 1 tablespoon raisins (optional)
- 1/4 teaspoon ground cinnamon

## *Procedure:*

1. In a saucepan, combine cooked rice and almond milk.
2. Stir in raisins and cinnamon.
3. Cook on low heat until the mixture thickens.
4. Serve warm or chilled.

## *Nutritional Content (per serving):*

- Calories: 220
- Protein: 5g
- Carbohydrates: 45g
- Fat: 3g
- Fiber: 2g

# 12. Cottage Cheese and Pineapple Bowl

## *Ingredients:*

- 1/2 cup cottage cheese
- 1/2 cup diced pineapple
- 1 tablespoon chopped almonds

## *Procedure*:

1. Place cottage cheese in a bowl.
2. Top with diced pineapple and chopped almonds.
3. Mix before eating.

## *Nutritional Content (per serving):*

- Calories: 180
- Protein: 14g
- Carbohydrates: 20g
- Fat: 6g
- Fiber: 2g

# 13. Mashed Sweet Potato Toast

## *Ingredients:*

- 1 slice whole grain bread, toasted
- 1/2 cup mashed sweet potato
- Dash of cinnamon

## *Procedure:*

1. Spread mashed sweet potato on the toasted bread.
2. Sprinkle a dash of cinnamon on top.
3. Enjoy as an open-faced toast.

## Nutritional Content (per serving):

- Calories: 210
- Protein: 4g
- Carbohydrates: 40g
- Fat: 2g
- Fiber: 6g

## 14. Soft Scrambled Egg with Avocado

*Ingredients:*

- 2 eggs

- 1/4 avocado, sliced

- Salt and pepper to taste

*Procedure*:

1. Scramble eggs in a pan over low heat until soft and creamy.

2. Serve with sliced avocado.

3. Season with salt and pepper.

*Nutritional Content (per serving):*

- Calories: 260

- Protein: 14g

- Carbohydrates: 8g

- Fat: 20g

- Fiber: 4g

## 15. Rice Cake with Almond Butter and Berries

### *Ingredients*:

- 1 rice cake
- 1 tablespoon almond butter
- Handful of mixed berries

### *Procedure*:

1. Spread almond butter on the rice cake.
2. Top with mixed berries.
3. Enjoy as a light and crunchy breakfast option.

### *Nutritional Content (per serving):*

- Calories: 190
- Protein: 5g
- Carbohydrates: 25g
- Fat: 8g
- Fiber: 4g

# 16. Pumpkin Spice Smoothie

## *Ingredients:*

- 1/2 cup canned pumpkin puree
- 1/2 cup Greek yogurt
- 1/2 cup almond milk
- 1 tablespoon honey
- Dash of pumpkin spice

## *Procedure:*

1. Blend pumpkin puree, Greek yogurt, almond milk, honey, and pumpkin spice until smooth.
2. Serve chilled.

## *Nutritional Content (per serving):*

- Calories: 220
- Protein: 14g
- Carbohydrates: 30g
- Fat: 5g
- Fiber: 6g

# 17. Spinach and Feta Omelette

## Ingredients:

- 2 eggs
- Handful of fresh spinach
- 2 tablespoons crumbled feta cheese
- Salt and pepper to taste

## Procedure:

1. Beat eggs in a bowl and season with salt and pepper.
2. Cook spinach in a pan until wilted, then pour in beaten eggs.
3. Sprinkle feta cheese over the omelette.
4. Cook until eggs are set and fold the omelette.
5. Serve hot.

## Nutritional Content (per serving):

- Calories: 250
- Protein: 18g
- Carbohydrates: 4g
- Fat: 18g
- Fiber: 1g

# 18. Blueberry Almond Smoothie

## Ingredients:

- 1/2 cup frozen blueberries
- 1/4 cup Greek yogurt
- 1/4 cup almond milk
- 1 tablespoon almond butter
- 1 teaspoon honey (optional)

## Procedure:

1. Blend frozen blueberries, Greek yogurt, almond milk, almond butter, and honey until smooth.
2. Serve immediately.

## Nutritional Content (per serving):

- Calories: 210
- Protein: 9g
- Carbohydrates: 25g
- Fat: 9g
- Fiber: 5g

# 19. Banana Walnut Overnight Oats

***Ingredients:***

- 1/2 cup rolled oats
- 1/2 cup almond milk
- 1/2 ripe banana, mashed
- 1 tablespoon chopped walnuts

***Procedure:***

1. Mix rolled oats, almond milk, mashed banana, and chopped walnuts in a jar.
2. Refrigerate overnight.
3. Enjoy cold in the morning.

***Nutritional Content (per serving):***

- Calories: 270
- Protein: 8g
- Carbohydrates: 35g
- Fat: 11g
- Fiber: 6g

# 20. Soft Boiled Quail Eggs with Toast Points

*Ingredients:*

- 4 quail eggs

- 1 slice whole grain bread, toasted and sliced into points

- Salt and pepper to taste

*Procedure:*

1. Boil quail eggs for 2-3 minutes for a soft-boiled consistency.

2. Serve with toasted bread points.

3. Season with salt and pepper.

*Nutritional Content (per serving):*

- Calories: 180

- Protein: 10g

- Carbohydrates: 20g

- Fat: 7g

- Fiber: 3g

# 21. Apple Cinnamon Breakfast Quinoa

*Ingredients*:

- 1/2 cup cooked quinoa
- 1/2 apple, diced
- 1 tablespoon chopped pecans
- Dash of cinnamon

*Procedure:*

1. Mix cooked quinoa, diced apple, chopped pecans, and cinnamon in a bowl.
2. Warm the mixture in a saucepan until the apple softens.
3. Serve warm.

*Nutritional Content (per serving):*

- Calories: 240
- Protein: 6g
- Carbohydrates: 40g
- Fat: 7g
- Fiber: 6g

# 22. Ricotta Cheese and Honey Toast

## *Ingredients:*

- 1 slice whole grain bread, toasted
- 1/4 cup ricotta cheese
- 1 tablespoon honey

## *Procedure:*

1. Spread ricotta cheese on the toasted bread.
2. Drizzle honey on top.
3. Enjoy as a creamy and sweet breakfast option.

## *Nutritional Content (per serving):*

- Calories: 220
- Protein: 9g
- Carbohydrates: 30g
- Fat: 7g
- Fiber: 3g

# 23. Soft Polenta with Berries

## *Ingredients:*

- 1/2 cup cooked polenta
- Handful of mixed berries
- 1 tablespoon maple syrup

## *Procedure:*

1. Cook polenta according to package instructions.
2. Serve with mixed berries on top.
3. Drizzle with maple syrup before serving.

## *Nutritional Content (per serving):*

- Calories: 210
- Protein: 4g
- Carbohydrates: 45g
- Fat: 2g
- Fiber: 5g

# 24. Turkey and Cheese Breakfast Wrap

## *Ingredients:*

- 1 whole grain tortilla
- 2 slices turkey
- 1 slice cheese (cheddar or Swiss)
- Handful of baby spinach leaves

## *Procedure:*

1. Layer turkey, cheese, and spinach on the tortilla.
2. Roll the tortilla and serve.

## *Nutritional Content (per serving):*

- Calories: 280
- Protein: 20g
- Carbohydrates: 25g
- Fat: 12g
- Fiber: 4g

## 25. Pumpkin Banana Muffins

*Ingredients*:

- 1/2 cup canned pumpkin puree
- 1 ripe banana, mashed
- 1 cup oat flour
- 1/4 cup honey or maple syrup
- 1 teaspoon baking powder

*Procedure:*

1. Preheat oven to 350°F (175°C).
2. Mix pumpkin puree, mashed banana, oat flour, honey or maple syrup, and baking powder in a bowl.
3. Pour the batter into muffin cups and bake for 20-25 minutes.
4. Allow to cool before serving.

*Nutritional Content (per serving - 1 muffin):*

- Calories: 120
- Protein: 3g
- Carbohydrates: 25g
- Fat: 1g
- Fiber: 3g

# 26. Soft Cornbread with Jam

## Ingredients:

- 1 slice cornbread, toasted
- 1 tablespoon fruit jam (e.g., raspberry or strawberry)

## Procedure:

1. Toast the cornbread until warm.
2. Spread jam on top and enjoy as a comforting breakfast option.

## Nutritional Content (per serving):

- Calories: 180
- Protein: 3g
- Carbohydrates: 35g
- Fat: 4g
- Fiber: 2g

# 27. Creamy Rice Cereal with Almond Butter

## *Ingredients*:

- 1/2 cup cooked rice cereal
- 2 tablespoons almond butter
- 1 tablespoon honey (optional)

## *Procedure*:

1. Mix cooked rice cereal and almond butter in a bowl.
2. Drizzle with honey if desired.
3. Serve warm.

## *Nutritional Content (per serving):*

- Calories: 270
- Protein: 7g
- Carbohydrates: 35g
- Fat: 11g
- Fiber: 3g

# 28. Soft Fruit Salad

*Ingredients*:

- 1/2 cup diced ripe melon (e.g., cantaloupe or honeydew)
- 1/2 cup diced ripe pear
- 1/2 cup ripe banana slices

*Procedure*:

1. Mix diced melon, pear, and banana in a bowl.
2. Serve as a refreshing and gentle breakfast option.

*Nutritional Content (per serving):*

- Calories: 150
- Protein: 2g
- Carbohydrates: 40g
- Fat: 0.5g
- Fiber: 6g

## 29. Soft Baked Apple with Cinnamon

*Ingredients*:

- 1 apple, cored
- 1 teaspoon cinnamon
- 1 tablespoon honey

*Procedure*:

1. Preheat oven to 350°F (175°C).
2. Place cored apple on a baking sheet and sprinkle with cinnamon.
3. Bake for 20-25 minutes until the apple softens.
4. Drizzle with honey before serving.

*Nutritional Content (per serving):*

- Calories: 100
- Protein: 0.5g
- Carbohydrates: 30g
- Fat: 0.5g
- Fiber: 5g

# 30. Soft Boiled Salmon with Rice

*Ingredients*:

- 1/2 cup cooked rice
- 2 oz. cooked soft-boiled salmon fillet
- Fresh dill for garnish

*Procedure:*

1. Place cooked rice on a plate.
2. Top with soft-boiled salmon fillet.
3. Garnish with fresh dill.

*Nutritional Content (per serving):*

- Calories: 290
- Protein: 22g
- Carbohydrates: 25g
- Fat: 11g
- Fiber: 1g

# *2.2 Delicious Lunch*

## 1. Turkey and Vegetable Soup

***Ingredients*:**

- 1 cup shredded turkey (cooked)

- 1 carrot, diced

- 1 celery stalk, diced

- 2 cups low-sodium chicken broth

- Salt and pepper to taste

***Procedure*:**

1. In a pot, combine shredded turkey, diced carrot, celery, and chicken broth.

2. Simmer over medium heat until vegetables are tender.

3. Season with salt and pepper.

4. Serve warm.

***Nutritional Content (per serving):***

- Calories: 200

- Protein: 20g

- Carbohydrates: 10g

- Fat: 8g

- Fiber: 2g

## 2. Soft Tofu and Spinach Salad

*Ingredients***:**

- 1/2 block soft tofu, cubed
- Handful of baby spinach leaves
- 1 tablespoon olive oil
- 1 tablespoon balsamic vinegar

*Procedure:*

1. Toss cubed tofu and baby spinach in a bowl.
2. Drizzle with olive oil and balsamic vinegar.
3. Gently mix before serving.

*Nutritional Content (per serving):*

- Calories: 180
- Protein: 12g
- Carbohydrates: 6g
- Fat: 12g
- Fiber: 2g

## 3. Mashed Potato and Chicken Casserole

*Ingredients:*

- 1 cup mashed potatoes
- 1 cup shredded chicken (cooked)
- 1/4 cup low-fat sour cream
- 1/4 cup shredded cheese (optional)

*Procedure:*

1. Preheat oven to 375°F (190°C).
2. In a baking dish, layer mashed potatoes, shredded chicken, and sour cream.
3. Sprinkle with shredded cheese if desired.
4. Bake for 20-25 minutes until heated through.

*Nutritional Content (per serving):*

- Calories: 250
- Protein: 18g
- Carbohydrates: 15g
- Fat: 12g
- Fiber: 2g

# 4. Soft Scrambled Eggs and Avocado Toast

## *Ingredients*:

- 2 eggs
- 1/4 avocado, sliced
- 1 slice whole grain bread, toasted

## *Procedure:*

1. Scramble eggs in a pan over low heat until soft.
2. Spread avocado slices on toasted bread.
3. Top with scrambled eggs and serve.

## *Nutritional Content (per serving):*

- Calories: 280
- Protein: 14g
- Carbohydrates: 20g
- Fat: 16g
- Fiber: 6g

# 5. Salmon and Quinoa Salad

## *Ingredients*:

- 4 oz. cooked salmon fillet, flaked
- 1/2 cup cooked quinoa
- Handful of mixed greens
- 1 tablespoon olive oil
- 1 tablespoon lemon juice

## *Procedure*:

1. Toss flaked salmon, cooked quinoa, and mixed greens in a bowl.
2. Drizzle with olive oil and lemon juice.
3. Mix gently before serving.

## *Nutritional Content (per serving):*

- Calories: 300
- Protein: 20g
- Carbohydrates: 20g
- Fat: 15g
- Fiber: 4g

## 6. Soft Chicken and Rice Congee

*Ingredients***:**

- 1/2 cup cooked white rice
- 1 cup shredded chicken (cooked)
- 3 cups low-sodium chicken broth
- Green onions for garnish
- Salt and pepper to taste

*Procedure:*

1. In a pot, combine cooked rice, shredded chicken, and chicken broth.
2. Simmer over low heat until the mixture thickens to a porridge-like consistency.
3. Season with salt and pepper.
4. Garnish with chopped green onions before serving.

*Nutritional Content (per serving):*

- Calories: 240
- Protein: 18g
- Carbohydrates: 25g
- Fat: 8g
- Fiber: 1g

## 7. Soft Turkey and Cheese Quesadilla

### *Ingredients*:

- 1 whole grain tortilla
- 1/4 cup shredded turkey (cooked)
- 1/4 cup shredded cheese (cheddar or mozzarella)
- Sliced bell peppers (optional)

### *Procedure*:

1. Place shredded turkey and shredded cheese on one half of the tortilla.
2. Add sliced bell peppers if desired.
3. Fold the tortilla in half.
4. Heat in a pan until the cheese melts and tortilla crisps slightly.
5. Serve warm.

### *Nutritional Content (per serving):*

- Calories: 280
- Protein: 18g
- Carbohydrates: 20g
- Fat: 14g
- Fiber: 3g

# 8. Soft Tuna Salad Sandwich

## *Ingredients*:

- 1/2 cup canned tuna, drained
- 1 tablespoon low-fat mayonnaise
- 1 teaspoon lemon juice
- 2 slices whole grain bread

## *Procedure*:

1. In a bowl, mix canned tuna, mayonnaise, and lemon juice.
2. Spread the tuna salad between two slices of bread.
3. Enjoy as a soft sandwich option.

## *Nutritional Content (per serving):*

- Calories: 260
- Protein: 20g
- Carbohydrates: 25g
- Fat: 9g
- Fiber: 5g

# 9. Soft Egg Salad Lettuce Wraps

## *Ingredients*:

- 2 hard-boiled eggs, mashed
- 1 tablespoon low-fat Greek yogurt
- Dash of mustard (optional)
- Lettuce leaves for wrapping

## *Procedure*:

1. Mix mashed hard-boiled eggs, Greek yogurt, and mustard in a bowl.
2. Spoon the egg salad into lettuce leaves.
3. Wrap and enjoy.

## *Nutritional Content (per serving):*

- Calories: 190
- Protein: 14g
- Carbohydrates: 5g
- Fat: 12g
- Fiber: 1g

# 10. Soft Meatball Soup

## *Ingredients:*

- 4 soft meatballs (chicken or turkey)
- 2 cups low-sodium chicken broth
- 1 carrot, sliced
- 1 celery stalk, diced
- Salt and pepper to taste

## *Procedure:*

1. In a pot, combine chicken broth, sliced carrot, diced celery, and soft meatballs.
2. Simmer over low heat until vegetables are tender and meatballs are heated through.
3. Season with salt and pepper.
4. Serve warm.

## *Nutritional Content (per serving):*

- Calories: 220
- Protein: 20g
- Carbohydrates: 10g
- Fat: 10g
- Fiber: 2g

## 11. Soft Veggie Rice Bowl

***Ingredients*:**

- 1/2 cup cooked white rice
- 1/2 cup soft-cooked vegetables (zucchini, carrots, bell peppers)
- 2 tablespoons hummus
- Fresh parsley for garnish

*Procedure:*

1. Place cooked rice in a bowl.
2. Top with soft-cooked vegetables and a dollop of hummus.
3. Garnish with fresh parsley before serving.

*Nutritional Content (per serving):*

- Calories: 230
- Protein: 6g
- Carbohydrates: 40g
- Fat: 5g
- Fiber: 6g

# 12. Soft Chicken and Vegetable Stir-Fry

## *Ingredients:*

- 1 cup shredded chicken (cooked)
- 1 cup soft-cooked vegetables (broccoli, snap peas, carrots)
- 1 tablespoon low-sodium soy sauce
- 1 teaspoon sesame oil
- Cooked rice for serving

## *Procedure:*

1. In a pan, stir-fry shredded chicken and soft-cooked vegetables with soy sauce and sesame oil.
2. Serve over cooked rice.

## *Nutritional Content (per serving):*

- Calories: 280
- Protein: 20g
- Carbohydrates: 25g
- Fat: 10g
- Fiber: 5g

## 13. Soft Lentil Soup

### *Ingredients:*

- 1/2 cup cooked lentils
- 2 cups low-sodium vegetable broth
- 1 carrot, diced
- 1 celery stalk, diced
- Salt and pepper to taste

### *Procedure:*

1. In a pot, combine cooked lentils, vegetable broth, diced carrot, and diced celery.
2. Simmer over low heat until vegetables are tender.
3. Season with salt and pepper.
4. Serve warm.

### *Nutritional Content (per serving):*

- Calories: 240
- Protein: 15g
- Carbohydrates: 40g
- Fat: 1g
- Fiber: 15g

# 14. Soft Tofu and Rice Noodles

## *Ingredients:*

- 1/2 cup soft tofu, cubed
- 1 cup cooked rice noodles
- 1/4 cup low-sodium broth (vegetable or chicken)
- 1 tablespoon chopped scallions
- 1 teaspoon sesame seeds (optional)

## *Procedure:*

1. Toss soft tofu and cooked rice noodles in a bowl.
2. Warm the broth in a pan and pour over the tofu and noodles.
3. Garnish with chopped scallions and sesame seeds.
4. Serve warm.

## *Nutritional Content (per serving):*

- Calories: 220
- Protein: 12g
- Carbohydrates: 35g
- Fat: 4g
- Fiber: 2g

# 15. Soft Turkey and Spinach Wrap

## Ingredients:

- 1 whole grain tortilla
- 1/4 cup shredded turkey (cooked)
- Handful of baby spinach leaves
- 1 tablespoon low-fat cream cheese

## Procedure:

1. Spread cream cheese on the tortilla.
2. Layer shredded turkey and baby spinach leaves.
3. Wrap and serve.

## Nutritional Content (per serving):

- Calories: 250
- Protein: 18g
- Carbohydrates: 25g
- Fat: 10g
- Fiber: 4g

# 16. Soft Baked Cod with Steamed Vegetables

## *Ingredients:*

- 4 oz. baked cod fillet
- 1 cup soft-steamed vegetables (cauliflower, carrots, green beans)
- Lemon wedge for garnish

## *Procedure:*

1. Bake the cod fillet until tender.
2. Steam the vegetables until soft.
3. Serve the cod with steamed vegetables and a lemon wedge.

## *Nutritional Content (per serving):*

- Calories: 230
- Protein: 25g
- Carbohydrates: 10g
- Fat: 5g
- Fiber: 5g

# 17. Soft Quinoa and Black Bean Salad

## *Ingredients:*

- 1/2 cup cooked quinoa
- 1/2 cup canned black beans, drained and rinsed
- 1/4 cup diced tomatoes
- 1 tablespoon chopped cilantro
- 1 tablespoon lime juice

## *Procedure:*

1. Mix cooked quinoa, black beans, diced tomatoes, chopped cilantro, and lime juice in a bowl.
2. Serve chilled or at room temperature.

## *Nutritional Content (per serving):*

- Calories: 240
- Protein: 10g
- Carbohydrates: 40g
- Fat: 3g
- Fiber: 10g

# 18. Soft Chicken and Mushroom Risotto

## *Ingredients:*

- 1/2 cup cooked Arborio rice
- 1/2 cup shredded chicken (cooked)
- 1/4 cup soft-cooked mushrooms
- 2 tablespoons low-sodium chicken broth
- Fresh parsley for garnish

## *Procedure:*

1. Combine cooked Arborio rice, shredded chicken, soft-cooked mushrooms, and chicken broth in a pan.
2. Cook over low heat until heated through.
3. Garnish with fresh parsley before serving.

## *Nutritional Content (per serving):*

- Calories: 260
- Protein: 18g
- Carbohydrates: 30g
- Fat: 7g
- Fiber: 2g

# 19. Soft Egg and Vegetable Frittata

## *Ingredients:*

- 2 eggs
- Handful of soft-cooked vegetables (bell peppers, onions, spinach)
- 1 tablespoon shredded cheese (optional)
- Salt and pepper to taste

## *Procedure:*

1. Whisk eggs in a bowl and mix in soft-cooked vegetables and shredded cheese.
2. Pour the mixture into a pan over low heat.
3. Cook until the eggs are set.
4. Season with salt and pepper.
5. Serve warm.

## *Nutritional Content (per serving):*

- Calories: 230
- Protein: 14g
- Carbohydrates: 5g
- Fat: 16g
- Fiber: 2g

## 20. Soft Beef and Potato Stew

### *Ingredients:*

- 4 oz. cooked beef, diced
- 1 cup soft-cooked potatoes
- 1 cup low-sodium beef broth
- 1 carrot, sliced
- Salt and pepper to taste

### *Procedure:*

1. Combine cooked beef, soft-cooked potatoes, sliced carrot, and beef broth in a pot.
2. Simmer over low heat until vegetables are tender and flavors combine.
3. Season with salt and pepper.
4. Serve warm.

### *Nutritional Content (per serving):*

- Calories: 270
- Protein: 20g
- Carbohydrates: 25g
- Fat: 10g
- Fiber: 3g

# 21. Soft Shrimp and Quinoa Stir-Fry

## Ingredients:

- 4 oz. cooked shrimp
- 1/2 cup cooked quinoa
- 1/2 cup soft-cooked mixed vegetables (bell peppers, broccoli, carrots)
- 1 tablespoon low-sodium soy sauce
- 1 teaspoon sesame oil

## Procedure:

1. In a pan, stir-fry cooked shrimp and soft-cooked vegetables with cooked quinoa, soy sauce, and sesame oil.
2. Cook until heated through and flavors meld.
3. Serve warm.

## Nutritional Content (per serving):

- Calories: 280
- Protein: 22g
- Carbohydrates: 30g
- Fat: 8g
- Fiber: 5g

# 22. Soft Pork and Rice Congee

*Ingredients:*

- 1/2 cup cooked white rice
- 4 oz. cooked pork, shredded
- 3 cups low-sodium pork or chicken broth
- Green onions for garnish
- Salt and pepper to taste

*Procedure:*

1. In a pot, combine cooked rice, shredded pork, and broth.
2. Simmer over low heat until the mixture thickens to a porridge-like consistency.
3. Season with salt and pepper.
4. Garnish with chopped green onions before serving.

*Nutritional Content (per serving):*

- Calories: 260
- Protein: 20g
- Carbohydrates: 25g
- Fat: 9g
- Fiber: 1g

# 23. Soft Turkey and Lentil Salad

*Ingredients:*

- 1/2 cup cooked lentils
- 1/2 cup shredded turkey (cooked)
- Handful of mixed greens
- 1 tablespoon balsamic vinaigrette

*Procedure:*

1. Toss cooked lentils, shredded turkey, and mixed greens in a bowl.
2. Drizzle with balsamic vinaigrette.
3. Mix gently before serving.

*Nutritional Content (per serving):*

- Calories: 240
- Protein: 18g
- Carbohydrates: 25g
- Fat: 8g
- Fiber: 6g

# 24. Soft Beef and Vegetable Stir-Fry

## Ingredients:

- 4 oz. cooked beef strips
- 1 cup soft-cooked mixed vegetables (bell peppers, snow peas, carrots)
- 1 tablespoon low-sodium teriyaki sauce
- Cooked rice for serving

## Procedure:

1. In a pan, stir-fry cooked beef strips and soft-cooked vegetables with teriyaki sauce.
2. Cook until heated through.
3. Serve over cooked rice.

## Nutritional Content (per serving):

- Calories: 270
- Protein: 22g
- Carbohydrates: 30g
- Fat: 7g
- Fiber: 4g

## 25. Soft Egg Drop Soup

### *Ingredients:*

- 2 eggs, beaten
- 3 cups low-sodium chicken broth
- Green onions for garnish
- Salt and pepper to taste

### *Procedure:*

1. In a pot, bring chicken broth to a gentle simmer.
2. Slowly pour beaten eggs into the simmering broth while stirring gently.
3. Cook for a minute until eggs are set.
4. Season with salt and pepper.
5. Garnish with chopped green onions before serving.

### *Nutritional Content (per serving):*

- Calories: 180
- Protein: 15g
- Carbohydrates: 5g
- Fat: 10g
- Fiber: 1g

# 26. Soft Chicken and Sweet Potato Mash

## Ingredients:

- 4 oz. cooked chicken breast, shredded
- 1/2 cup soft-cooked sweet potato mash
- 1 tablespoon low-sodium chicken broth
- Fresh parsley for garnish

## Procedure:

1. In a bowl, mix shredded chicken, sweet potato mash, and chicken broth.
2. Warm in the microwave or on the stovetop until heated through.
3. Garnish with fresh parsley before serving.

## Nutritional Content (per serving):

- Calories: 240
- Protein: 20g
- Carbohydrates: 25g
- Fat: 6g
- Fiber: 4g

# 27. Soft Tuna and Avocado Salad

*Ingredients:*

- 1/2 cup canned tuna, drained
- 1/2 avocado, mashed
- Handful of mixed greens
- 1 tablespoon olive oil
- 1 tablespoon lemon juice

*Procedure:*

1. In a bowl, mix canned tuna, mashed avocado, mixed greens, olive oil, and lemon juice.
2. Toss gently before serving.

*Nutritional Content (per serving):*

- Calories: 250
- Protein: 18g
- Carbohydrates: 15g
- Fat: 15g
- Fiber: 8g

## 28. Soft Beef and Barley Stew

### Ingredients:

- 4 oz. cooked beef, diced
- 1/2 cup cooked barley
- 2 cups low-sodium beef broth
- 1 carrot, sliced
- Salt and pepper to taste

### Procedure:

1. In a pot, combine cooked beef, cooked barley, sliced carrot, and beef broth.
2. Simmer over low heat until vegetables are tender and flavors meld.
3. Season with salt and pepper.
4. Serve warm.

### Nutritional Content (per serving):

- Calories: 280
- Protein: 20g
- Carbohydrates: 30g
- Fat: 8g
- Fiber: 6g

# 29. Soft Vegetable and Bean Soup

## *Ingredients:*

- 1 cup soft-cooked mixed vegetables (zucchini, squash, tomatoes)
- 1/2 cup canned beans (kidney beans, black beans)
- 2 cups low-sodium vegetable broth
- Fresh herbs for garnish
- Salt and pepper to taste

## *Procedure:*

1. In a pot, combine soft-cooked vegetables, canned beans, and vegetable broth.
2. Simmer over low heat until flavors meld.
3. Season with salt and pepper.
4. Garnish with fresh herbs before serving.

## *Nutritional Content (per serving):*

- Calories: 220
- Protein: 10g
- Carbohydrates: 40g
- Fat: 1g
- Fiber: 12g

# 30. Soft Tofu and Tomato Salad

## *Ingredients:*

- 1/2 cup soft tofu, cubed
- 1/2 cup diced tomatoes
- 1 tablespoon balsamic vinaigrette
- Fresh basil for garnish

## *Procedure:*

1. Mix cubed soft tofu and diced tomatoes in a bowl.
2. Drizzle with balsamic vinaigrette.
3. Garnish with fresh basil before serving.

## *Nutritional Content (per serving):*

- Calories: 200
- Protein: 12g
- Carbohydrates: 15g
- Fat: 10g
- Fiber: 5g

# *2.3 Gastroparesis-Friendly Dinner Recipes*

## 1. Soft Chicken and Rice Casserole

*Ingredients*:

- 1 cup cooked white rice
- 1 cup shredded chicken (cooked)
- 1/2 cup soft-cooked vegetables (peas, carrots)
- 1/4 cup low-fat cream of mushroom soup
- Salt and pepper to taste

*Procedure:*

1. Preheat oven to 375°F (190°C).
2. In a baking dish, layer cooked rice, shredded chicken, soft-cooked vegetables, and cream of mushroom soup.
3. Bake for 20-25 minutes until heated through.

*Nutritional Content (per serving):*

- Calories: 280
- Protein: 20g
- Carbohydrates: 30g
- Fat: 8g
- Fiber: 3g

## 2. Soft Salmon and Quinoa Bowl

*Ingredients:*

- 4 oz. baked salmon fillet, flaked
- 1/2 cup cooked quinoa
- 1/2 cup soft-cooked mixed vegetables (zucchini, bell peppers)
- 1 tablespoon olive oil
- 1 tablespoon lemon juice

*Procedure:*

1. Arrange flaked salmon, cooked quinoa, and soft-cooked mixed vegetables in a bowl.
2. Drizzle with olive oil and lemon juice.
3. Serve warm.

*Nutritional Content (per serving):*

- Calories: 320
- Protein: 25g
- Carbohydrates: 30g
- Fat: 12g
- Fiber: 6g

## 3. Soft Turkey Meatballs with Mashed Potatoes

### *Ingredients:*

- 4 soft turkey meatballs
- 1/2 cup mashed potatoes
- 1/4 cup low-sodium turkey gravy
- Fresh parsley for garnish

### *Procedure:*

1. Warm soft turkey meatballs and mashed potatoes.
2. Place mashed potatoes on a plate and top with warmed meatballs.
3. Drizzle with turkey gravy.
4. Garnish with fresh parsley before serving.

### *Nutritional Content (per serving):*

- Calories: 300
- Protein: 20g
- Carbohydrates: 25g
- Fat: 12g
- Fiber: 3g

## 4. Soft Baked Chicken and Sweet Potato Mash

*Ingredients:*

- 4 oz. baked chicken breast, diced
- 1/2 cup soft-cooked sweet potato mash
- 1 tablespoon low-sodium chicken broth
- Fresh herbs for garnish

*Procedure:*

1. In a bowl, mix diced baked chicken, sweet potato mash, and chicken broth.
2. Warm in the microwave or on the stovetop until heated through.
3. Garnish with fresh herbs before serving.

*Nutritional Content (per serving):*

- Calories: 280
- Protein: 22g
- Carbohydrates: 25g
- Fat: 9g
- Fiber: 4g

## 5. Soft Beef Stew with Soft Cooked Vegetables

*Ingredients:*

- 4 oz. cooked beef cubes
- 1 cup soft-cooked mixed vegetables (carrots, green beans, potatoes)
- 1 cup low-sodium beef broth
- Salt and pepper to taste

*Procedure:*

1. Combine cooked beef cubes, soft-cooked mixed vegetables, and beef broth in a pot.
2. Simmer over low heat until flavors meld and vegetables are tender.
3. Season with salt and pepper before serving.

*Nutritional Content (per serving):*

- Calories: 300
- Protein: 24g
- Carbohydrates: 20g
- Fat: 12g
- Fiber: 4g

## 6. Soft Tofu Stir-Fry with Rice

*Ingredients:*

- 1/2 cup soft tofu cubes
- 1 cup soft-cooked mixed vegetables (broccoli, bell peppers, mushrooms)
- 1 tablespoon low-sodium soy sauce
- 1 teaspoon sesame oil
- Cooked rice for serving

*Procedure:*

1. Stir-fry soft tofu and soft-cooked mixed vegetables in a pan with soy sauce and sesame oil.
2. Cook until heated through and flavors meld.
3. Serve over cooked rice.

*Nutritional Content (per serving):*

- Calories: 260
- Protein: 16g
- Carbohydrates: 30g
- Fat: 9g
- Fiber: 5g

# 7. Soft Lentil Chili

## *Ingredients:*

- 1/2 cup cooked lentils
- 1/2 cup soft-cooked diced tomatoes
- 1/4 cup diced onions
- 1 teaspoon chili powder
- Salt and pepper to taste

## *Procedure:*

1. Combine cooked lentils, soft-cooked diced tomatoes, diced onions, chili powder, salt, and pepper in a pot.
2. Simmer over low heat until flavors meld.
3. Serve warm.

## *Nutritional Content (per serving):*

- Calories: 240
- Protein: 14g
- Carbohydrates: 40g
- Fat: 1g
- Fiber: 16g

# 8. Soft Baked Cod with Soft Steamed Vegetables

*Ingredients:*

- 4 oz. baked cod fillet
- 1 cup soft-steamed mixed vegetables (cauliflower, carrots, green beans)
- Lemon wedge for garnish

*Procedure*:

1. Bake the cod fillet until tender.
2. Steam mixed vegetables until soft.
3. Serve the cod with steamed vegetables and a lemon wedge.

*Nutritional Content (per serving):*

- Calories: 250
- Protein: 26g
- Carbohydrates: 15g
- Fat: 8g
- Fiber: 6g

## 9. Soft Eggplant and Tomato Bake

*Ingredients:*

- 1 small eggplant, sliced and soft-baked
- 1/2 cup soft-cooked diced tomatoes
- 1/4 cup shredded cheese (optional)
- Fresh basil for garnish

*Procedure:*

1. Layer soft-baked eggplant slices and soft-cooked diced tomatoes in a baking dish.
2. Optionally, sprinkle with shredded cheese.
3. Bake until heated through and cheese melts.
4. Garnish with fresh basil before serving.

*Nutritional Content (per serving):*

- Calories: 220
- Protein: 8g
- Carbohydrates: 20g
- Fat: 12g
- Fiber: 8g

# 10. Soft Chicken and Vegetable Curry

*Ingredients:*

- 4 oz. cooked chicken, diced
- 1/2 cup soft-cooked mixed vegetables (peas, carrots, potatoes)
- 1/4 cup coconut milk
- 1 tablespoon curry powder
- Cooked rice for serving

*Procedure:*

1. In a pan, combine diced cooked chicken, soft-cooked mixed vegetables, coconut milk, and curry powder.
2. Simmer until heated through and flavors meld.
3. Serve over cooked rice.

*Nutritional Content (per serving):*

- Calories: 290
- Protein: 22g
- Carbohydrates: 25g
- Fat: 10g
- Fiber: 4g

## 11. Soft Turkey and Vegetable Stir-Fry

### *Ingredients:*

- 1 cup shredded turkey (cooked)
- 1 cup soft-cooked mixed vegetables (bell peppers, snap peas, carrots)
- 1 tablespoon low-sodium soy sauce
- 1 teaspoon sesame oil
- Cooked rice for serving

### *Procedure:*

1. In a pan, stir-fry shredded turkey and soft-cooked mixed vegetables with soy sauce and sesame oil.
2. Cook until heated through.
3. Serve over cooked rice.

### *Nutritional Content (per serving):*

- Calories: 270
- Protein: 18g
- Carbohydrates: 30g
- Fat: 8g
- Fiber: 5g

# 12. Soft Shrimp and Brown Rice Pilaf

## *Ingredients:*

- 4 oz. cooked shrimp
- 1/2 cup cooked brown rice
- 1/2 cup soft-cooked mixed vegetables (broccoli, bell peppers)
- 1 tablespoon olive oil
- 1 tablespoon lemon juice

## *Procedure:*

1. Combine cooked shrimp, cooked brown rice, and soft-cooked mixed vegetables in a pan.
2. Drizzle with olive oil and lemon juice.
3. Heat until warmed through.
4. Serve warm.

## *Nutritional Content (per serving):*

- Calories: 290
- Protein: 20g
- Carbohydrates: 30g
- Fat: 10g
- Fiber: 6g

## 13. Soft Tuna and Quinoa Salad

*Ingredients:*

- 1/2 cup canned tuna, drained
- 1/2 cup cooked quinoa
- 1/4 cup diced cucumbers
- 1 tablespoon low-fat vinaigrette

*Procedure:*

1. Mix canned tuna, cooked quinoa, and diced cucumbers in a bowl.
2. Drizzle with low-fat vinaigrette.
3. Serve chilled or at room temperature.

*Nutritional Content (per serving):*

- Calories: 250
- Protein: 22g
- Carbohydrates: 25g
- Fat: 8g
- Fiber: 4g

## 14. Soft Chicken and Broccoli Casserole

### *Ingredients:*

- 1 cup shredded chicken (cooked)
- 1 cup soft-cooked broccoli florets
- 1/4 cup low-fat cream of chicken soup
- Salt and pepper to taste

### *Procedure:*

1. Preheat oven to 375°F (190°C).
2. In a baking dish, layer shredded chicken, soft-cooked broccoli, and cream of chicken soup.
3. Bake for 20-25 minutes until heated through.

### *Nutritional Content (per serving):*

- Calories: 280
- Protein: 20g
- Carbohydrates: 20g
- Fat: 10g
- Fiber: 4g

# 15. Soft Egg Drop Stir-Fry

*Ingredients:*

- 2 eggs, beaten
- 1 cup soft-cooked mixed vegetables (peas, carrots, bell peppers)
- 1 tablespoon low-sodium soy sauce
- Cooked rice for serving

*Procedure:*

1. Stir-fry soft-cooked mixed vegetables in a pan with low-sodium soy sauce.
2. Pour beaten eggs over the vegetables while stirring gently until eggs are set.
3. Serve over cooked rice.

*Nutritional Content (per serving):*

- Calories: 260
- Protein: 16g
- Carbohydrates: 30g
- Fat: 9g
- Fiber: 4g

# 16. Soft Beef and Mushroom Stroganoff

## *Ingredients:*

- 4 oz. cooked beef strips
- 1/2 cup soft-cooked mushrooms
- 1/4 cup low-fat sour cream
- Cooked egg noodles for serving

## *Procedure:*

1. In a pan, combine cooked beef strips, soft-cooked mushrooms, and low-fat sour cream.
2. Warm until heated through.
3. Serve over cooked egg noodles.

## *Nutritional Content (per serving):*

- Calories: 300
- Protein: 22g
- Carbohydrates: 25g
- Fat: 10g
- Fiber: 3g

## 17. Soft Chicken and Cauliflower Rice

### *Ingredients:*

- 4 oz. cooked chicken breast, shredded
- 1 cup soft-cooked cauliflower rice
- 1/4 cup low-sodium chicken broth
- Fresh parsley for garnish

### *Procedure:*

1. Mix shredded cooked chicken, soft-cooked cauliflower rice, and chicken broth in a pan.
2. Warm until heated through.
3. Garnish with fresh parsley before serving.

### *Nutritional Content (per serving):*

- Calories: 280
- Protein: 24g
- Carbohydrates: 15g
- Fat: 10g
- Fiber: 4g

## 18. Soft Turkey and Sweet Potato Mash

### *Ingredients:*

- 4 oz. shredded cooked turkey
- 1/2 cup soft-cooked sweet potato mash
- 1 tablespoon low-sodium turkey gravy
- Fresh herbs for garnish

### *Procedure:*

1. In a bowl, mix shredded cooked turkey and soft-cooked sweet potato mash.
2. Warm in the microwave or on the stovetop until heated through.
3. Drizzle with low-sodium turkey gravy.
4. Garnish with fresh herbs before serving.

### *Nutritional Content (per serving):*

- Calories: 290
- Protein: 20g
- Carbohydrates: 25g
- Fat: 10g
- Fiber: 4g

# 19. Soft Lentil and Vegetable Curry

## *Ingredients:*

- 1/2 cup cooked lentils
- 1 cup soft-cooked mixed vegetables (cauliflower, peas, carrots)
- 1/4 cup coconut milk
- 1 tablespoon curry powder
- Cooked rice for serving

## *Procedure:*

1. Combine cooked lentils, soft-cooked mixed vegetables, coconut milk, and curry powder in a pan.
2. Simmer until heated through and flavors meld.
3. Serve over cooked rice.

## *Nutritional Content (per serving):*

- Calories: 260
- Protein: 14g
- Carbohydrates: 30g
- Fat: 10g
- Fiber: 8g

## 20. Soft Chicken and Spinach Pasta

### *Ingredients:*

- 4 oz. cooked chicken, diced
- 1 cup soft-cooked spinach
- 1/2 cup cooked pasta
- 1 tablespoon olive oil
- Fresh basil for garnish

### *Procedure:*

1. In a pan, combine diced cooked chicken, soft-cooked spinach, cooked pasta, and olive oil.
2. Heat until warmed through.
3. Garnish with fresh basil before serving.

### *Nutritional Content (per serving):*

- Calories: 280
- Protein: 20g
- Carbohydrates: 25g
- Fat: 10g
- Fiber: 4g

## 21. Soft Beef and Vegetable Skewers

### *Ingredients:*

- 4 oz. cooked beef chunks
- 1 cup soft-cooked bell peppers, onions, and cherry tomatoes
- 1 tablespoon low-sodium teriyaki sauce
- Cooked rice for serving

### *Procedure:*

1. Skewer cooked beef chunks and soft-cooked vegetables.
2. Grill or broil until heated through.
3. Brush with teriyaki sauce while cooking.
4. Serve over cooked rice.

### *Nutritional Content (per serving):*

- Calories: 290
- Protein: 22g
- Carbohydrates: 30g
- Fat: 8g
- Fiber: 4g

# 22. Soft Turkey and Rice Pilaf

## *Ingredients:*

- 4 oz. cooked turkey, shredded
- 1/2 cup cooked brown rice
- 1/2 cup soft-cooked mixed vegetables (peas, carrots)
- 1 tablespoon low-sodium chicken broth
- Fresh herbs for garnish

## *Procedure:*

1. Combine shredded cooked turkey, cooked brown rice, soft-cooked mixed vegetables, and chicken broth in a pan.
2. Warm until heated through.
3. Garnish with fresh herbs before serving.

## *Nutritional Content (per serving):*

- Calories: 280
- Protein: 20g
- Carbohydrates: 25g
- Fat: 9g
- Fiber: 4g

# 23. Soft Tofu and Vegetable Stir-Fry

## *Ingredients:*

- 1/2 cup soft tofu cubes
- 1 cup soft-cooked mixed vegetables (broccoli, snap peas, bell peppers)
- 1 tablespoon low-sodium soy sauce
- 1 teaspoon sesame oil
- Cooked rice for serving

## *Procedure*:

1. Stir-fry soft tofu and soft-cooked mixed vegetables in a pan with soy sauce and sesame oil.
2. Cook until heated through and flavors meld.
3. Serve over cooked rice.

## *Nutritional Content (per serving):*

- Calories: 260
- Protein: 16g
- Carbohydrates: 30g
- Fat: 9g
- Fiber: 5g

## 24. Soft Chicken and Rice Soup

*Ingredients:*

- 4 oz. shredded cooked chicken
- 1/2 cup soft-cooked rice
- 2 cups low-sodium chicken broth
- 1 carrot, diced
- Salt and pepper to taste

*Procedure:*

1. Combine shredded cooked chicken, soft-cooked rice, diced carrot, and chicken broth in a pot.
2. Simmer over low heat until flavors meld and vegetables are tender.
3. Season with salt and pepper before serving.

*Nutritional Content (per serving):*

- Calories: 270
- Protein: 20g
- Carbohydrates: 25g
- Fat: 8g
- Fiber: 3g

# 25. Soft Turkey and Potato Bake

## *Ingredients:*

- 4 oz. cooked turkey, shredded
- 1/2 cup soft-cooked diced potatoes
- 1/4 cup low-fat shredded cheese
- Fresh parsley for garnish

## *Procedure:*

1. Layer shredded cooked turkey and soft-cooked diced potatoes in a baking dish.
2. Sprinkle with low-fat shredded cheese.
3. Bake until heated through and cheese melts.
4. Garnish with fresh parsley before serving.

## *Nutritional Content (per serving):*

- Calories: 280
- Protein: 20g
- Carbohydrates: 25g
- Fat: 9g
- Fiber: 4g

# 26. Soft Beef and Quinoa Stuffed Peppers

## *Ingredients:*

- 4 oz. cooked ground beef
- 1/2 cup cooked quinoa
- 2 soft-cooked bell peppers
- 1/4 cup low-sodium tomato sauce
- Fresh herbs for garnish

## *Procedure:*

1. Mix cooked ground beef and cooked quinoa.
2. Stuff soft-cooked bell peppers with the beef and quinoa mixture.
3. Top with low-sodium tomato sauce.
4. Bake until heated through.
5. Garnish with fresh herbs before serving.

## *Nutritional Content (per serving):*

- Calories: 290
- Protein: 22g
- Carbohydrates: 25g
- Fat: 9g
- Fiber: 5g

# 27. Soft Chicken and Rice Casserole

## *Ingredients*:

- 1 cup shredded cooked chicken
- 1/2 cup soft-cooked rice
- 1/4 cup low-fat cream of chicken soup
- Salt and pepper to taste

## *Procedure*:

1. Preheat oven to 375°F (190°C).
2. In a baking dish, combine shredded cooked chicken, soft-cooked rice, and cream of chicken soup.
3. Bake for 20-25 minutes until heated through.

## *Nutritional Content (per serving)*:

- Calories: 280
- Protein: 20g
- Carbohydrates: 20g
- Fat: 10g
- Fiber: 3g

# 28. Soft Tuna and Brown Rice Salad

## *Ingredients:*

- 1/2 cup canned tuna, drained
- 1/2 cup cooked brown rice
- 1/4 cup diced cucumbers
- 1 tablespoon low-fat vinaigrette

## *Procedure:*

1. Mix canned tuna, cooked brown rice, and diced cucumbers in a bowl.
2. Drizzle with low-fat vinaigrette.
3. Serve chilled or at room temperature.

## *Nutritional Content (per serving):*

- Calories: 260
- Protein: 20g
- Carbohydrates: 25g
- Fat: 8g
- Fiber: 4g

# 29. Soft Turkey and Vegetable Soup

## *Ingredients:*

- 4 oz. shredded cooked turkey
- 1 cup soft-cooked mixed vegetables (corn, green beans, carrots)
- 2 cups low-sodium turkey broth
- Salt and pepper to taste

## *Procedure:*

1. Combine shredded cooked turkey, soft-cooked mixed vegetables, and turkey broth in a pot.
2. Simmer over low heat until flavors meld.
3. Season with salt and pepper before serving.

## *Nutritional Content (per serving):*

- Calories: 280
- Protein: 22g
- Carbohydrates: 20g
- Fat: 9g
- Fiber: 4g

# 30. Soft Eggplant and Zucchini Bake

## *Ingredients:*

- 1 small eggplant, sliced and soft-baked
- 1/2 cup soft-cooked sliced zucchini
- 1/4 cup shredded cheese (optional)
- Fresh basil for garnish

## *Procedure:*

1. Layer soft-baked eggplant slices and soft-cooked sliced zucchini in a baking dish.
2. Optionally, sprinkle with shredded cheese.
3. Bake until heated through and cheese melts.
4. Garnish with fresh basil before serving.

## *Nutritional Content (per serving):*

- Calories: 220
- Protein: 8g
- Carbohydrates: 20g
- Fat: 12g
- Fiber: 8g

# 2.4 Gastroparesis-Friendly Snack and Dessert Recipes

## 1. Soft Banana Oat Cookies

### Ingredients:

- 2 ripe bananas, mashed
- 1 cup rolled oats
- 1/4 cup chopped nuts or seeds (optional)
- Cinnamon to taste

### Procedure:

1. Preheat oven to 350°F (175°C).
2. Mix mashed bananas, rolled oats, chopped nuts/seeds, and cinnamon in a bowl.
3. Spoon mixture onto a baking sheet lined with parchment paper.
4. Bake for 12-15 minutes until set.

### Nutritional Content (per serving - 2 cookies):

- Calories: 120
- Protein: 3g
- Carbohydrates: 20g
- Fat: 4g
- Fiber: 3g

## 2. Soft Berry Smoothie Bowl

### *Ingredients:*

- 1 cup frozen mixed berries
- 1 ripe banana
- 1/2 cup yogurt (or dairy-free alternative)
- 2 tablespoons honey (optional)
- Toppings: sliced bananas, nuts, seeds

### *Procedure:*

1. Blend frozen berries, banana, yogurt, and honey until smooth.
2. Pour into a bowl and top with sliced bananas, nuts, or seeds.

***Nutritional Content:*** *(Nutritional values may vary based on toppings used)*

## 3. Soft Baked Apples

### *Ingredients:*

- 2 apples, cored and sliced
- 1 tablespoon honey
- 1 teaspoon cinnamon
- 1 tablespoon chopped nuts

### *Procedure:*

1. Preheat oven to 350°F (175°C).
2. Place apple slices in a baking dish, drizzle with honey, and sprinkle with cinnamon and nuts.
3. Bake for 15-20 minutes until apples are soft.

### *Nutritional Content (per serving - 1 apple):*

- Calories: 80
- Protein: 1g
- Carbohydrates: 20g
- Fat: 2g
- Fiber: 4g

# 4. Soft Yogurt Parfait

## *Ingredients:*

- 1 cup Greek yogurt (or dairy-free alternative)
- 1/4 cup granola (low-fat and low-sugar)
- 1/2 cup soft-cooked fruit (berries, peaches)
- Honey or maple syrup for sweetness (optional)

## *Procedure:*

1. Layer yogurt, granola, and soft-cooked fruit in a glass or bowl.
2. Drizzle with honey or maple syrup if desired.

*Nutritional Content (per serving): (Nutritional values may vary based on granola used)*

## 5. Soft Pumpkin Pudding

*Ingredients:*

- 1 cup canned pumpkin puree
- 1/2 cup Greek yogurt (or dairy-free alternative)
- 2 tablespoons honey or maple syrup
- 1 teaspoon pumpkin pie spice

*Procedure:*

1. Mix pumpkin puree, Greek yogurt, honey/maple syrup, and pumpkin pie spice in a bowl until smooth.
2. Refrigerate for at least 30 minutes before serving.

*Nutritional Content (per serving):*

- Calories: 90
- Protcin: 4g
- Carbohydrates: 15g
- Fat: 2g
- Fiber: 4g

# 6. Soft Rice Pudding

*Ingredients:*

- 1 cup cooked white rice
- 1 cup almond milk (or any preferred milk)
- 2 tablespoons honey or maple syrup
- 1 teaspoon vanilla extract
- Cinnamon for garnish

*Procedure:*

1. In a saucepan, combine cooked rice, almond milk, honey/maple syrup, and vanilla extract.
2. Simmer over low heat until thickened.
3. Sprinkle with cinnamon before serving.

*Nutritional Content (per serving):*

- Calories: 150
- Protein: 2g
- Carbohydrates: 30g
- Fat: 2g
- Fiber: 1g

# 7. Soft Peanut Butter and Banana Rice Cakes

*Ingredients:*

- Rice cakes
- Peanut butter (smooth)
- Sliced bananas
- Honey (optional)

*Procedure:*

1. Spread peanut butter on rice cakes.
2. Top with sliced bananas.
3. Drizzle with honey if desired.

**Nutritional Content (per serving - 2 rice cakes):** *(Values may vary based on peanut butter and honey used)*

# 8. Soft Avocado Chocolate Mousse

## Ingredients:

- 2 ripe avocados
- 1/4 cup cocoa powder
- 1/4 cup honey or maple syrup
- 1 teaspoon vanilla extract

## Procedure:

1. Blend avocados, cocoa powder, honey/maple syrup, and vanilla extract until smooth.
2. Chill in the refrigerator for at least 1 hour before serving.

## Nutritional Content (per serving):

- Calories: 200
- Protein: 3g
- Carbohydrates: 25g
- Fat: 13g
- Fiber: 8g

## 9. Soft Fruit Salad

*Ingredients:*

- Soft-cooked mixed fruits (berries, peaches, kiwi)
- 1 tablespoon honey or lemon juice (optional)
- Fresh mint leaves for garnish

*Procedure:*

1. Mix soft-cooked mixed fruits in a bowl.
2. Drizzle with honey or lemon juice if desired.
3. Garnish with fresh mint leaves.

***Nutritional Content (per serving):*** *(Nutritional values may vary based on fruits used)*

# 10. Soft Chia Seed Pudding

## *Ingredients:*

- 1/4 cup chia seeds
- 1 cup almond milk (or any preferred milk)
- 1 tablespoon honey or maple syrup
- 1/2 teaspoon vanilla extract

## *Procedure:*

1. Mix chia seeds, almond milk, honey/maple syrup, and vanilla extract in a bowl.
2. Refrigerate overnight or for at least 4 hours until thickened.

## *Nutritional Content (per serving):*

- Calories: 120
- Protein: 3g
- Carbohydrates: 15g
- Fat: 5g
- Fiber: 7g

# 11. Soft Baked Pear with Cinnamon

## *Ingredients:*

- 2 ripe pears, halved and cored
- 1 tablespoon honey
- 1 teaspoon cinnamon

## *Procedure:*

1. Preheat oven to 375°F (190°C).
2. Place pear halves on a baking sheet, drizzle with honey, and sprinkle with cinnamon.
3. Bake for 20-25 minutes until pears are soft.

## *Nutritional Content (per serving - 1 pear):*

- Calories: 90
- Protein: 1g
- Carbohydrates: 25g
- Fat: 0g
- Fiber: 6g

## 12. Soft Mango Yogurt Popsicles

*Ingredients:*

- 1 cup diced mango
- 1 cup Greek yogurt (or dairy-free alternative)
- 2 tablespoons honey or agave syrup

*Procedure:*

1. Blend diced mango, Greek yogurt, and honey/agave syrup until smooth.
2. Pour mixture into popsicle molds and freeze until set.

*Nutritional Content (per serving - 1 popsicle): (Values may vary based on popsicle mold size)*

# 13. Soft Cinnamon Baked Sweet Potatoes

## Ingredients:

- 2 sweet potatoes, sliced
- 1 tablespoon melted coconut oil
- 1 teaspoon cinnamon
- Honey for drizzling (optional)

## Procedure:

1. Preheat oven to 400°F (200°C).
2. Toss sweet potato slices in melted coconut oil and cinnamon.
3. Bake for 20-25 minutes until soft.
4. Drizzle with honey if desired before serving.

## Nutritional Content (per serving - 1 sweet potato):

- Calories: 100
- Protein: 2g
- Carbohydrates: 25g
- Fat: 2g
- Fiber: 4g

# 14. Soft Blueberry Chia Jam

## *Ingredients:*

- 1 cup fresh or frozen blueberries
- 2 tablespoons chia seeds
- 1 tablespoon honey or maple syrup

## *Procedure:*

1. In a saucepan, cook blueberries over low heat until they start to break down.
2. Mash blueberries with a fork and stir in chia seeds and honey/maple syrup.
3. Cook for another 5 minutes until thickened.
4. Allow to cool before serving.

***Nutritional Content (per serving):*** *(Values may vary based on serving size)*

# 15. Soft Peanut Butter and Jelly Sandwiches

## Ingredients:

- Soft bread slices
- Peanut butter (smooth)
- Low-sugar jelly or jam

## Procedure:

1. Spread peanut butter on one bread slice and jelly/jam on another.
2. Combine both slices to make a sandwich.

## Nutritional Content (per serving - 1 sandwich):

*(Values may vary based on bread and toppings used)*

# 16. Soft Baked Banana with Cinnamon

## *Ingredients:*

- 2 ripe bananas
- Cinnamon to sprinkle

## *Procedure:*

1. Preheat oven to 350°F (175°C).
2. Place whole bananas (with skin) on a baking sheet.
3. Bake for 15-20 minutes until bananas are soft.
4. Sprinkle with cinnamon before serving.

## *Nutritional Content (per serving - 1 banana):*

- Calories: 90
- Protein: 1g
- Carbohydrates: 23g
- Fat: 0g
- Fiber: 3g

# 17. Soft Carrot Cake Bites

## *Ingredients:*

- 1 cup grated carrots
- 1/2 cup almond flour
- 1/4 cup shredded coconut
- 2 tablespoons honey
- 1 teaspoon cinnamon

## *Procedure:*

1. Mix grated carrots, almond flour, shredded coconut, honey, and cinnamon in a bowl.
2. Form into small bite-sized balls.
3. Refrigerate for 30 minutes before serving.

## *Nutritional Content (per serving - 2 bites):*

- Calories: 90
- Protein: 2g
- Carbohydrates: 12g
- Fat: 4g
- Fiber: 2g

# 18. Soft Yogurt Bark

## *Ingredients:*

- 1 cup Greek yogurt (or dairy-free alternative)
- 1/4 cup soft-cooked fruit (berries, mango)
- 2 tablespoons honey or maple syrup
- Nuts or seeds for topping

## *Procedure:*

1. Mix Greek yogurt, soft-cooked fruit, and honey/maple syrup in a bowl.
2. Spread the mixture evenly on a parchment-lined baking sheet.
3. Sprinkle with nuts or seeds.
4. Freeze until set, then break into pieces before serving.

***Nutritional Content (per serving - 1 piece):*** *(Values may vary based on toppings used)*

## 19. Soft Rice Cake with Cottage Cheese and Berries

*Ingredients:*

- Rice cakes

- Cottage cheese (soft or blended)

- Fresh berries

*Procedure:*

1. Spread cottage cheese on rice cakes.

2. Top with fresh berries.

*Nutritional Content (per serving - 2 rice cakes): (Values may vary based on cottage cheese and berries used)*

# 20. Soft Chocolate Chia Pudding

*Ingredients:*

- 1/4 cup chia seeds
- 1 cup almond milk (or any preferred milk)
- 2 tablespoons cocoa powder
- 2 tablespoons honey or maple syrup

*Procedure:*

1. Mix chia seeds, almond milk, cocoa powder, and honey/maple syrup in a bowl.
2. Refrigerate overnight or for at least 4 hours until thickened.

*Nutritional Content:*

*(Values may vary based on cottage cheese and berries used)*

# Chapter 3: Advanced Cooking Techniques

## 3.1 Advanced Recipe Modifications

Creating delicious meals while considering dietary restrictions or health conditions often involves modifications to traditional recipes. Advanced recipe modifications offer a gateway to explore culinary creativity, adapting dishes to meet specific nutritional needs or accommodate health challenges like gastroparesis. This guide delves into advanced techniques, empowering you to craft flavorful and nourishing meals tailored to individual preferences and requirements.

### Understanding Recipe Modifications

Modifying recipes goes beyond simple ingredient substitutions. It encompasses an understanding of ingredients, their roles in cooking, and the impact alterations may have on taste, texture, and nutritional value. It's an art form requiring attention to detail and an understanding of how flavors and components interact.

### Adapting for Gastroparesis

Gastroparesis demands specialized dietary adjustments. Traditional recipes often contain ingredients challenging for sensitive stomachs. Advanced modifications involve replacing hard-to-digest elements with softer, gentler alternatives. For instance, opting for soft-cooked vegetables, lean meats, or easily digestible grains can transform a dish into a gastroparesis-friendly delight.

## Balancing Flavor and Nutrition

Maintaining flavor while modifying recipes is crucial. Ingredients like herbs, spices, citrus zest, and vinegars can enhance taste without adding unnecessary elements. Nutritional balance remains pivotal, ensuring meals are rich in essential nutrients without compromising digestibility. Incorporating high-protein, low-fat options or nutrient-dense vegetables ensures recipes remain both flavorful and healthful.

## Techniques for Modification

- **Texture Alterations**: Achieving the desired texture often involves innovative techniques. Blending, mashing, or slow-cooking ingredients can transform dishes into softer, easily digestible delights.
- **Ingredient Substitutions**: Substituting ingredients requires a keen understanding of their roles. Opting for easily digestible alternatives, such as replacing regular flour with almond or oat flour, can revolutionize recipes.
- **Portion Control:** Adjusting portion sizes can impact digestibility. Smaller, more frequent meals distributed throughout the day can aid digestion for individuals with gastroparesis.
- **Cooking Methods**: Experimenting with different cooking methods—steaming, stewing, or braising—can influence digestibility while intensifying flavors.

## Customizing Recipes

Advanced modifications encourage customization. Personalizing recipes by adjusting spice levels, incorporating varied cooking fats, or altering seasoning combinations caters to individual taste preferences. Furthermore, exploring ethnic cuisines and their traditional adaptations offers a treasure trove of innovative cooking techniques and flavor profiles.

Mastering advanced recipe modifications demands patience, experimentation, and an understanding of ingredients and their interactions. It's a journey toward crafting delectable, health-conscious meals tailored to specific needs, ensuring that each dish remains both a culinary delight and a nourishing experience.

**DR. BENJAMIN THOMPSON**

# 3 .2 Incorporating Medicinal Ingredients

Gastroparesis, characterized by delayed stomach emptying, presents unique dietary challenges. Exploring the integration of medicinal ingredients into gastroparesis-friendly recipes can offer therapeutic benefits, aiding digestion and easing symptoms. This comprehensive guide delves into the realm of medicinal ingredients, their properties, and their incorporation into culinary practices, empowering individuals to manage gastroparesis through nourishing, therapeutic meals.

## Understanding Medicinal Ingredients

Medicinal ingredients encompass a diverse array of herbs, spices, and natural substances known for their therapeutic properties. From aiding digestion to reducing inflammation and easing discomfort, these elements play a pivotal role in traditional medicine and holistic healing practices.

## Properties Beneficial for Gastroparesis

1. **Digestive Aids:** Certain ingredients possess digestive-boosting properties. Ginger, for example, is renowned for its ability to soothe the digestive system and alleviate nausea, making it a valuable addition to gastroparesis-friendly recipes.

2. **Anti-inflammatory Agents:** Inflammation exacerbates gastroparesis symptoms. Turmeric, rich in curcumin, acts as a potent anti-inflammatory, potentially alleviating discomfort associated with inflammation.

3. **Calming Agents:** Chamomile and peppermint possess calming properties, soothing the stomach and reducing discomfort often experienced by individuals with gastroparesis.

4. **Antioxidants:** Ingredients like garlic, cinnamon, and green tea are rich in antioxidants, combating oxidative stress and supporting overall digestive health.

## Incorporating Medicinal Ingredients

1. **Herbs and Spices:** Infusing dishes with medicinal herbs and spices can elevate flavor while offering therapeutic benefits. Incorporating fresh or dried herbs like basil, thyme, and oregano, or spices such as cinnamon, cumin, and turmeric, introduces both taste and health-enhancing properties.

2. **Teas and Infusions:** Brewing herbal teas or infusions using calming herbs like chamomile or peppermint between meals can provide relief from discomfort, aiding in digestion.

3. **Supplements:** Consider incorporating supplements with medicinal properties. For instance, probiotics may promote gut health, aiding digestion and potentially alleviating gastroparesis symptoms.

4. **Natural Sweeteners:** Replacing refined sugars with natural sweeteners like honey or stevia not only enhances the nutritional value of dishes but also offers potential digestive benefits.

## Cooking Techniques

1. **Simmering and Steeping:** Slow-cooking techniques like simmering or steeping medicinal ingredients in broths or teas can maximize their therapeutic potential while infusing dishes with their properties.

2. **Balancing Flavors:** Experimenting with combinations of medicinal ingredients requires a delicate balance. Understanding their flavor profiles and complementary pairings ensures that therapeutic elements enhance rather than overpower the dish.

3. **Infusion in Cooking Fats:** Infusing medicinal ingredients like garlic or ginger in cooking oils can impart their health benefits into dishes, offering a subtle yet effective medicinal touch.

## Cautions and Considerations

1. **Allergies and Sensitivities:** Some individuals may have allergies or sensitivities to certain medicinal ingredients. It's crucial to be mindful and cautious when introducing new elements into diets.

2. **Dosage and Moderation:** While medicinal ingredients offer therapeutic benefits, moderation is key. Excessive consumption may lead to adverse effects or interactions with medications.

3. **Consultation with Healthcare Providers:** Consulting healthcare professionals or registered dietitians before incorporating medicinal ingredients is essential, especially for individuals managing specific health conditions or taking medications.

# Meet the Author: Benjamin Thompson

**Exploring the Author's Insights:**

Discover more about Benjamin Thompson's background, insights, and journey in health and culinary wellness through his Amazon Author Central page. Click the link or scan the QR code below to dive deeper into the author's profile, exploring an array of informative articles, author updates, and additional resources related to health, wellness, and culinary solutions.

Explore these captivating works by Benjamin Thompson, each offering unique perspectives on health, wellness, and the art of nourishing cuisine. Visit the Amazon Author Central page to access more captivating reads and engage with the author's enriching content.

**YOU CAN FOLLOW ACCOUNT SO YOU GET NOTIFIED WHEN WE DROP UPDATED AND NEW COOKBOOKS ON GOOD HEALTH.**

**CLICK LINK BELOW**

amazon.com/author/benjaminthompson

**OR**

# SCAN QR CODE

# *Other Works by Benjamin Thompson:*

Explore beyond "Nourishing Solutions" and delve into Benjamin Thompson's diverse collection of literature, encompassing a range of health-centric topics and culinary adventures. Here are two captivating books authored by Benjamin Thompson:

1. **" MODERN PIONEER COOKBOOK: Over 200 recipes of Farm-to-Table Flavors, Sustainable Eats, and Timeless Techniques for the Culinary Adventurer from a traditional foods kitchen**.

   Are you ready to embark on a culinary journey that marries the charm of yesteryears with the innovation of today's kitchens?

   "Modern Pioneer Cookbook" is your passport to a world of farm-to-table flavors, sustainable eats, and timeless techniques that will transform your cooking and reconnect you with the essence of pioneer living.

## Click on this link to view

https://www.amazon.com/MODERN-PIONEER-COOKBOOK-Farm-Table/dp/B0CJK4SQM9/ref=sr_1_5?Adv-Srch-Books-Submit.x=0&Adv-Srch-Books-Submit.y=0&qid=1704262149&refinements=p_27%3ADr.+benjamin+thompson&s=books&sr=1-5&unfiltered=1

or

## scan QR code to view

2. **" BREAST CANCER DIET COOKBOOK FOR BEGINNERS: 1500 days meal of complete Beginner's Guide to a Nourishing Breast Cancer fighting Diet for prevention, ... and Renewed Well-Being"**

Are you or a loved one facing the challenges of breast cancer?

Are you a newly diagnosed breast cancer patient searching for ways to support your health and well-being on your journey?"

### Click link to view

https://www.amazon.com/BREAST-CANCER-DIET-COOKBOOK-BEGINNERS/dp/B0CJ47N9Q4/ref=sr_1_1?Adv-Srch-Books-Submit.x=0&Adv-Srch-Books-Submit.y=0&qid=1704264224&refinements=p_27%3ADr.+benjamin+thompson&s=books&sr=1-1&unfiltered=1

### or

### scan QR code to view

Dive into the world of health, wellness, and flavorful culinary adventures with Benjamin Thompson's enlightening works!

# Summary and Conclusion

**"Nourishing Solutions: A Gastroparesis-Friendly Cookbook"**

In "Nourishing Solutions," we embarked on a culinary journey designed for individuals managing gastroparesis. This cookbook is a comprehensive compilation of gentle-on-the-stomach recipes, crafted meticulously to ensure both flavor and ease for those facing digestive challenges.

**What We've Explored:**

1. **Thorough Understanding:** We delved into the nuances of gastroparesis, exploring its impact on digestion, lifestyle, and dietary guidelines.

2. **Gastroparesis-Friendly Recipes:** Over 100 recipes were meticulously developed, spanning breakfast, lunch, dinner, snacks, and desserts. Each recipe focused on ingredients and cooking methods tailored to ease symptoms and foster a delightful dining experience.

3. **Advanced Techniques:** We delved into advanced modifications, empowering readers to adapt recipes to meet individual preferences and dietary needs, including the integration of medicinal ingredients for therapeutic benefits.

4. **30-Day Meal Plan:** A 30-day meal plan was meticulously curated, providing a diverse array of nourishing meals while considering dietary limitations and ensuring optimal digestion.

**Our Journey Doesn't End Here:**

As we conclude this culinary expedition, your feedback becomes invaluable. We invite you to share your experiences, thoughts, and suggestions for "Nourishing Solutions." Your reviews and insights will aid in crafting future editions, ensuring even more tailored, flavorful, and helpful recipes for individuals managing gastroparesis.

**DR. BENJAMIN THOMPSON** 

Your reviews will shape the future of this cookbook, helping us understand what worked well, what could be improved, and how we can better support you on your journey towards gastronomic wellness.

Thank you for joining us on this flavorful and nurturing adventure. We eagerly await your feedback as we continue to refine and enhance "Nourishing Solutions" to better serve you and those navigating the challenges of gastroparesis.

Savor the meals, embrace the flavors, and continue on your path to wellness through nourishing and satisfying cuisine.

Warm regards,

**[Benjamin Thompson]**

# NOTES